I0130816

TOOLS FOR SUCCESSFULLY TREATING Pain

IN MAINSTREAM MEDICINE

MARK YEZAK, B.S., D.C.

PHILOSOPHY TO SPINE TREATMENT

INTERNATIONAL HEALTH PUBLISHING
www.InternationalHealthPublishing.com

INTERNATIONAL HEALTH PUBLISHING
Established 2008
Publishing Group Affirming Truth & Innate Wisdom

Copyright © 2014 by MARK YEZAK, B.S., D.C.

All rights reserved, including the right of reproduction in whole or in part in any form or by any means, electronic or mechanical, including photocopy, recording, or any information storage and retrieval system, without written permission from the publisher, author, and copyright owners; except by a reviewer who may quote brief passages in review.

First International Health Publishing trade paperback edition August 2014.

For information about special discounts for bulk purchase, please write to writer@InternationalHealthPublishing.com.

International Health Publishing can bring authors to your live events. For more information or to book an event, contact writer@InternationalHealthPublishing.com or for more information visit us online: www.InternationalHealthPublishing.com.

The author of this book does not dispense medical advice or suggest the use of any technique as a form of treatment for physical, emotional, or medical problems without the advice of a qualified wellness professional, either directly or indirectly. In the event you use any of the information in this book, the author and the publisher are in no way liable for any misuse of material.

Tools for Successfully Treating Pain
In Mainstream Medicine

MARK YEZAK, B.S., D.C.

ISBN-13: 978-0-9857956-8-9

Library of Congress Control Number: 2014942365

SAN 856-6925

Manufactured in the United States of America, and printed on the finest
100% postconsumer-waste recycled paper

10 9 8 7 6 5 4 3 2 1

ACKNOWLEDGEMENTS

There are a number of individuals I thank for their direct and indirect involvement in this book. I offer my first heartfelt gratitude to my loving wife, Heather, and to my children Haley, Hayden and Hudson, who have always encouraged me to see the good in everyone and everything.

My deep appreciation goes out to my dedicated staff members Becky Sandefur and Becky Couch, who have helped me with this book and who have always stood by our practice and shown me what it means to have a staff with tremendous dedication.

Endless gratitude to my Partner Scott Neuburger DC for 18 great years together!

I am especially grateful for Monette Smith, our advertising executive who has always pushed to keep our creativity in the forefront.

Finally, many thanks must go to our extraordinary clients and my amazing team at HSRC who have dedicated their time and energy every day to changing the lives of others.

Houston Spine and Rehabilitation Centers (HSRC) are known regionally for helping people and relieving symptoms that vary from acute pain, musculoskeletal strains to failed surgeries with chronic pain. HSRC is built upon a platform of Customer Service that assists in the helping patients ultimately returning to their activities of daily living as quickly as possible. In doing this, we have established multi-disciplinary models of healthcare that offer our patients a variety of treatment options, as well as efficient and effective care.

This manual is written to provide a foundation for not only musculoskeletal pain management, but also to provide you with the resources we have developed to ensure a smooth patient process. You may notice many variations to each model within this manual. Every patient has different needs, schedules and financial ability. This training manual includes treatment options and financial processes that have proven to be effective and efficient for managing a successful multi-disciplinary practice.

LEGEND
Tool Shed = Office
Tools = Treatment/Techniques for Patient Care

Disclaimer: This manual is not a directive on how to treat patients, but rather a model for practice management. Every patient is evaluated and treated according to their needs. Doctors are to diagnose and treat patients according to the guidelines and scope of their practice. This manual does not supersede a doctor's judgment for treatment and patient care. This manual is to be used as a guide, a training source, and is written for educational purposes only.

TABLE OF CONTENTS

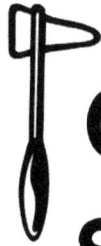**T**OOLS FOR SUCCESSFULLY TREATING 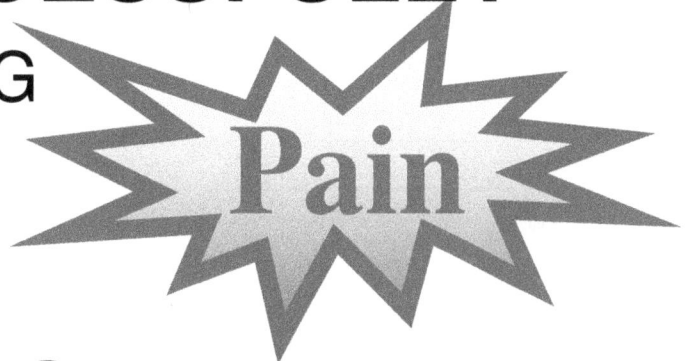**Pain**

IN **MAINSTREAM MEDICINE**

TOOLS
FOR EVERY
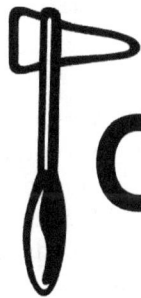
OOL SHED

A **multi-disciplinary healthcare practice** is a group of health care providers from different disciplines, each providing specific services to the patient under the same roof. Convenient and efficient, it's an approach to patient care involving more than one discipline that assists with maximizing effectiveness of care and providing positive outcomes.

Our multi-disciplinary team is composed of a select group of specialized doctors and therapists. With over 50 years of combined healthcare service experience, our team is able to draw from a wealth of knowledge and expertise in treating and preventing injuries, while also maximizing health. Our goal is to not only address individual conditions or injuries, but to educate our patients for the prevention of similar injuries in the future. To do this, we have carefully chosen the most effective treatments and specialized health professionals to deliver quality services to the people we serve.

THE 5 TOOLS IN YOUR TOOL SHED

1) Chiropractic
2) Physical Therapy
3) Pain Management
4) Traction
5) Surgery

CHIROPRACTIC

Over the last 20 years, the evolution of Chiropractic is significant. Just 15 years ago, Chiropractic doctors were considered 'outsiders' in the healthcare arena. This view was starting to transform as many great leading Doctors of Chiropractic emerged as qualified diagnosticians. They set the foundation for new role for chiropractors in mainstream healthcare. Doctors like Dennis Skogsberg, D.C., Jay Triano, D.C., and Bill Defoyd, D.C laid the groundwork for chiropractors as primary care neuro-musculoskeletal specialists. As many others, I was confused as a Chiropractor defining subluxation. Therefore, I took the base chiropractic model and, with the help of George Aubert, D.C., molded it to fit a successful practice model that meets patients where they are on the spectrum of health. Using the tools and techniques of the aforementioned specialty providers, I blended a perfect mixture. The model is arranged into three levels of care. While this does not cover all the minute variables – from symptoms to conditions – the model provides guidance in selecting modalities to best serve a patient. The treatment level options include a variety of tools to complete your tool belt and to apply according to patient needs.

PHYSICAL THERAPY

Hippocrates was an ancient Greek physician and often referred to as the father of western medicine. He is believed to have been the first practitioners of physical therapy, promoting massage, manual therapy techniques and hydrotherapy to treat people in 460 BC. Physical therapy as we know it today has been recognized since the end of the 19th century. After that time, American orthopedic surgeons hired women trained in physical education, massage, and remedial exercise to treat children with disabilities, and so it began.

Physical Therapy has a broad scope. When one envisions the use of PT they think of strengthening. However with spine care the real benefit is with the Stretching protocols. The addition of PT to my practice has been invaluable. By balancing the muscular system it allows chiropractic to further improve the function of the skeletal and nervous systems. Therefore, instead of focusing on one system, all are addressed and corrected.

VAX-D / SPINAL DECOMPRESSION TRACTION THERAPY PROTOCOL

Dr. Allan Dyer, PhD, MD originally developed and pioneered a non-surgical spinal decompression in 1985. In 1991, he then introduced the first non-surgical spinal decompression table known as Vax-D. It was controlled by a pneumatic system that progressively applied and released pressure to the spine. A traction force was applied to reduce nerve pressure, and release muscle guarding and spasm. Many other non-surgical spinal decompression tables have been developed with features believed to mimic or enhance the effectiveness of the original concept.

I found Vax-D in 2000 and began using it in my practice. A patient would say, "I feel that if I could just hang by my feet or be pulled apart and stretched, I would feel better." Of course you do. It feels great to unload all the stress and gravity from the spine. I have had amazing patient outcomes using the Vax-D traction model. I have helped thousands of people with back and neck pain. This led me to publish "Fountain of Youth for the Lower Back." Use traction when appropriate and you will be amazed.

PAIN MANAGEMENT

Pain management uses an interdisciplinary approach to assist in lessening or alleviating a patient's pain and helps improve a persons' quality of life. While pain usually resolves once the initial injury is treated and has had time to heal, it may need to be treated simultaneously with analgesic-type medications. Occasionally chronic pain management symptoms will need to be managed with a Pain Management team that may include Medical doctors, along with Chiropractors and Physical Therapists.

I personally suffer from back pain due to a large Lumbar HNP. Two years ago, Surgery was recommended but due to my profession and the stress I place on my own back every day, I elected to not have surgery. My only option was an Epidural Steroid Injection given by a pain management physician to reduce the severe leg pain and loss of function. Following my procedure, I was able to return to normal activity quickly with no side effects. I have seen similar recoveries many times with my patients. We have found by injecting the affected area and reducing a patient's pain without unnecessary Narcotics it allows people to more quickly engage in active care. This provides a better outcome and reduces the chance of chronic pain.

SURGERY

Surgery is the treatment of injuries or disorders of the body by incision or manipulation, especially with instruments. The oldest evidence-based operation was for Trepanation in which a hole is made into the skull to treat health problems related to intracranial pressure and other diseases. Since individuals first discovered how to make and use tools, they advanced their abilities to develop surgical techniques, each time more sophisticated than the last. Advances in these fields have converted surgery from a perilous "art" into a scientific specialty capable of improving and even alleviating many conditions.

Not everyone responds positively to conservative procedures; so don't expect this. Some conditions require surgery. Over the years I have sent numerous patients who have failed conservative care to surgery for various reasons – and generally the outcomes are positive. It's all about understanding your conservative options and choosing the patients so they obtain the desired outcome. There are many conservative surgeons who will make the final decision if they feel confident in a positive outcome. Don't hold on to the patient forever and hold them back when a surgical recommendation could be a savior in helping them recover.

APPLYING

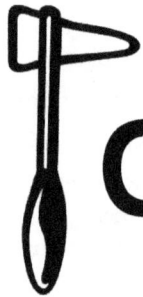 YOUR

TOOLS

WHEN TO USE YOUR TOOLS

Making a difference in peoples lives is a driving force for most healthcare professionals. Each person to enter your office will have different needs, and likely have different health goals. As a service provider, ultimately the target is to meet a person's individual needs and guide them towards their unique health objectives.

In our experience we have found a variety of treatment levels that facilitate successful outcomes. The level of treatment for each individual depends greatly upon a person's state of health when they arrive.

TREATMENT LEVELS

Initially patients are evaluated, or managed, according to current condition. Patients are counseled regarding their condition and provided a proposed treatment plan. HSRC uses the three models (levels) to describe treatment options. During the consultation the provider discusses options and determines a plan of care.

A patient's schedule and ability to commit to the plan is taken into consideration. Treatment initially begins with conservative methods (Level 1), and if indicated, progresses to more aggressive measures (Level 3). Levels of treatment are as follows:

- **THE CONSERVATIVE TREATMENT - LEVEL (1)** – Chiropractic Manipulation and Physical Therapy/Physical Medicine. This type of treatment is usually prescribed for (4-6 weeks.) Initially, acute patients are treated daily with modalities to calm inflammation. Pain Management options, more specifically consulting with a Pain Management Physician regarding medications, are recommended if a patient's pain level is elevated due to an inflammatory state. After the patient's symptoms begin to decrease and the patient is able to tolerate more manual treatment, manipulation and therapeutic stretching are performed. In addition, Physical Therapy is relative and a preferred treatment option that not only rehabilitates an injury, but also is used to strengthen core muscles and correct posture concerns. The use of both chiropractic and physical therapy is optimal to increase mechanical and functional levels simultaneously and can be performed on the same day.

  - o RED FLAGS - Severe radiculopathy and/or positive Neurological signs in this stage require immediate MRI or additional diagnostic studies.

- **INTERMEDIATE TREATMENT - LEVEL (2)** – This level is used for patients who have participated in the conservative option (Level 1) prior to presenting for their consultation, or have failed the conservative option in the recommended plan of care. If a patient has failed to improve using the conservative method, an MRI or other diagnostic testing should be ordered. Results are then reviewed and progressive options discussed based on the results of MRI. A non-surgical option is Traction (AKA Vax-D or Spinal Decompression), with or without injections. Traction is an effective treatment alternative for cervical or lumbar HNP's, disc degeneration, and mild neuro foraminal stenosis. The traction protocol is 25 consecutive visits combined with modality and therapeutic treatment. It is then followed by 4 weeks of Physical Therapy exercises to strengthen and improve musculoskeletal structure. Please be aware of contraindications, more specifically spinal stenosis.
  - o In Level 2, pain management injections can be implemented. Pain levels or radicular findings are always a deciding factor when adding pain management to a treatment plan.

Injections may be used in conjunction with traction at this level of treatment and are dependent upon the MRI findings in correlation with the exam.

NOTE: Injections are typically performed in a series of three. Two options are Epidural Steroid Injections (ESI) or Facet Injections, predicated on MRI and clinical findings. Injections do not have to be used only in conjunction with traction but may also be used as a sole remedy for relieving inflammation or radiculitis.

- **ADVANCED TREATMENT - LEVEL (3)** – This level of treatment is used when surgery is imminent or desired. If the patient fails or does not achieve desired level of improvement with both Levels 1 and 2, or presents with a structural concern they are referred to an orthopedic/neuro surgeon for a consultation. Patient is sent with all imaging and reports on file. The patients are scheduled for a follow-up appointment to discuss any surgical recommendations. In the event a surgical procedure is scheduled, the patient is scheduled to return to our office for rehabilitative therapy once released from surgical care. If surgery is not an option, an outside referral may be needed to recommend other maintenance and long-term options. There is great value in obtaining a surgeons' (or other specialists') opinion, as this practitioner may provide further options of care.

- **CHIROPRACTIC MANAGEMENT - LEVEL (4)** – This level of treatment is recommended to patients that have completed their plan of care successfully or present initially with manageable symptoms, posture or health concerns. Chiropractic care is designed to assist in managing pain and dysfunction caused by activities of daily living (traumas, thoughts, toxins), while also maximizing neurological function and overall health. Treatment is rendered for the patient's current health concerns or in accordance with any updates in their health since their last visit. This is sometimes a one-time visit for a single occurrence or a series of a few visits, and does not necessarily have to include a complete active treatment regimen. In the process of controlling their symptoms, patients are taught about the benefits of having regular chiropractic evaluations and treatments to avoid future reoccurrences and progression of degeneration, as well as to maximize their overall health.

The design is to establish a baseline and maintain the best health possible. Routine chiropractic care has proven effective for relieving pain, reducing arthritis, preventing injury, maintaining joint function, improving neurological function and optimizing health.

Patient education is an enormous part of patient management and is essential for their understanding of health and wellness.

HOME CARE RECOMMENDATIONS

In addition to in-office services, some patients may benefit from receiving instructions for home care. Most patients are willing to put in an extra effort to maximize their health benefits. Recommendations for home care may include a Work-Station Ergonomic Analysis and Correction, or even the development of a complete Home Exercise Program – with or without a personal trainer.

Other therapeutic products may be recommended to assist with improving the rate of healing and preventing injury, such as purchasing a new mattress or using specific pillows, posture supports, TENS Units, or other therapeutic devices. Again, patient education is key for their understanding and compliance.

TREATMENT FLOW

Evaluation Performed,
X-rays obtained &
diagnosis determined

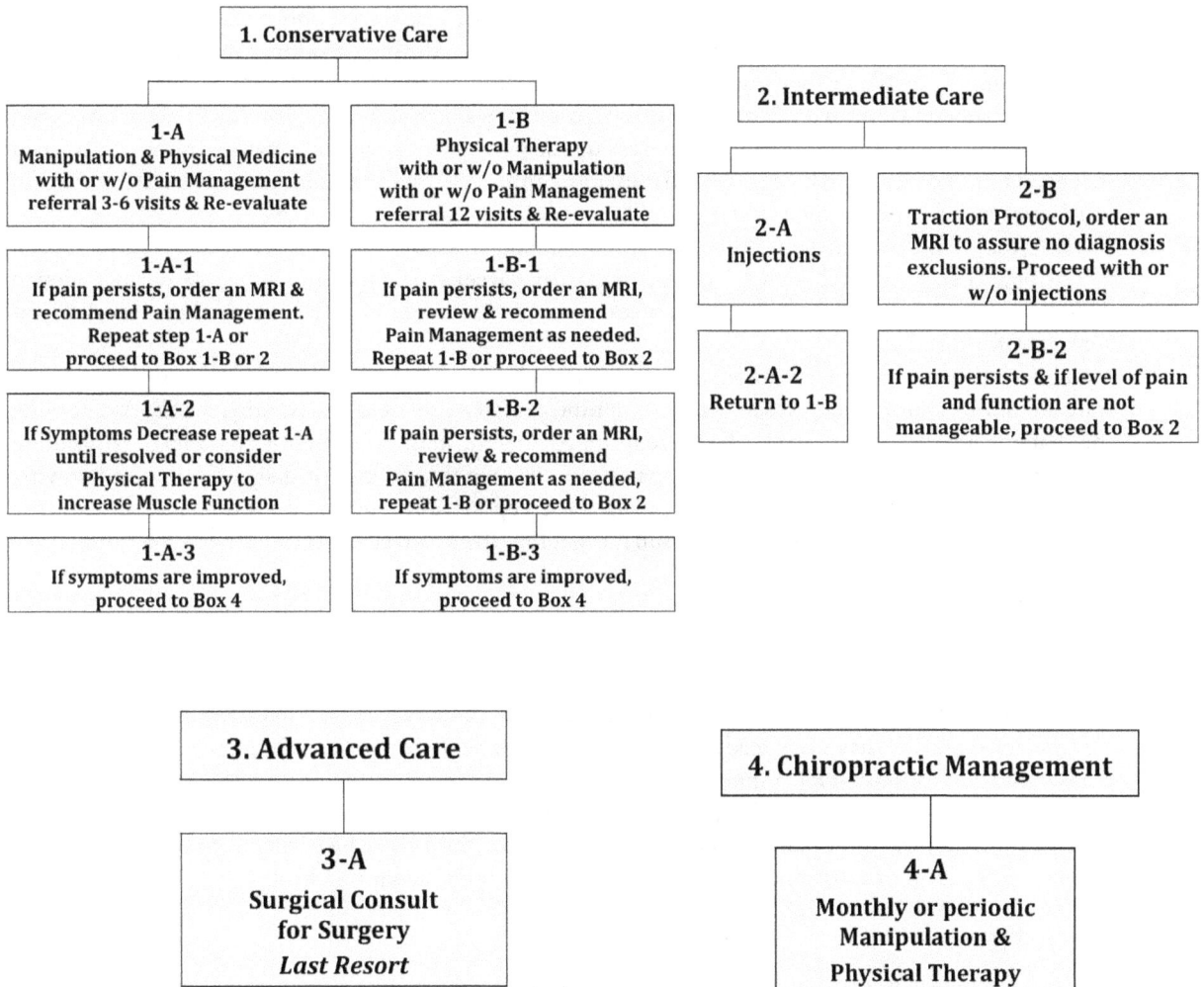

1. Conservative Care

1-A
Manipulation & Physical Medicine
with or w/o Pain Management
referral 3-6 visits & Re-evaluate

1-A-1
If pain persists, order an MRI &
recommend Pain Management.
Repeat step 1-A or
proceed to Box 1-B or 2

1-A-2
If Symptoms Decrease repeat 1-A
until resolved or consider
Physical Therapy to
increase Muscle Function

1-A-3
If symptoms are improved,
proceed to Box 4

1-B
Physical Therapy
with or w/o Manipulation
with or w/o Pain Management
referral 12 visits & Re-evaluate

1-B-1
If pain persists, order an MRI,
review & recommend
Pain Management as needed.
Repeat 1-B or proceeed to Box 2

1-B-2
If pain persists, order an MRI,
review & recommend
Pain Management as needed,
repeat 1-B or proceed to Box 2

1-B-3
If symptoms are improved,
proceed to Box 4

2. Intermediate Care

2-A
Injections

2-A-2
Return to 1-B

2-B
Traction Protocol, order an
MRI to assure no diagnosis
exclusions. Proceed with or
w/o injections

2-B-2
If pain persists & if level of pain
and function are not
manageable, proceed to Box 2

3. Advanced Care

3-A
Surgical Consult
for Surgery
Last Resort

4. Chiropractic Management

4-A
Monthly or periodic
Manipulation &
Physical Therapy

PROVEN TREATMENT PLANS

Every new patient receives a complete evaluation and diagnostic studies to establish their diagnosis and treatment recommendations. Within every level of care there are a variety of treatment options to include. One patient may benefit from a specific type of muscle therapy, while another may benefit from a different approach. Clinical indications dictate the course of action. Generally speaking, treatment plans typically begin with passive care and as a condition improves/stabilizes, transition into active therapy. In any case, the goal is to allow for improved activities of daily living, improved neurological function, and improved health.

LEVEL 1 - OPTIONS

- Patients in acute phase or initial treatment phase are treated daily for one week with modalities and/or manipulation. After one week of treatment they are reassessed and reduced to 2- 3 times a week for 2-3 weeks, depending on their specific needs. If they require rehabilitation or core strengthening to avoid further injury, patients are recommended for Physical Therapy. If a patient has pain that continues past 2 or 3 weeks or their condition digresses, an MRI is obtained and injections are discussed and ordered if necessary. A patient with radicular pain is referred for pain management in order to reduce acute inflammation and allow them to enter an active rehab program much earlier and expedite their outcome.
- Patients that don't present with acute symptoms yet still lack core strength are considered to engage in Physical Therapy and scheduled 3 times a week for 4 weeks. If a patient's schedule doesn't allow 3 days a week, then a schedule of 2 times a week for 6 weeks can be beneficial. One time a week is not sufficient for PT.
- Patients that have completed an acute therapy treatment or have completed Physical Therapy are transitioned to chiropractic care at a rate of 1 time per week or once every other week. At the time the patient reaches their level of desired improvement, they are then transitioned to routine chiropractic management, at a rate of once per month. Due to activities of daily life, time and gravity, the spine slowly compresses down (known as the creep effect); regular check-ups and adjustments promote healthy joints and neurological function, allow the synovial fluid to lubricate the joints, and reduce degenerative arthritis.

LEVEL 2 - OPTIONS

- Traction is used if a patient continues to have radicular pain and an MRI has been performed showing compression or HNP's. This treatment is a more aggressive method and used when manipulation and PT have not made improvement to patients symptoms. Patients are scheduled 25 consecutive days and then PT 3 times per week for 4 weeks to strengthen the core.
- Injections are a procedure to reduce swelling locally. Patient education is imperative to explain that injections are not simply a pain procedure but rather a method to reduce swelling and inflammation locally. Elimination of inflammation ideally increases the body's ability to heal.

LEVEL 3 - OPTIONS

- A Surgical consult is considered if a patient has failed conservative or invasive care. Additionally, patients that have any type of clinical contraindications for the use of conservative methods are directly referred prior to any in-office treatment. A surgical opinion is obtained when and if the following occur: neurological loss, failed conservative care, red flags or there is abnormal pathology.

LEVEL 4 - OPTIONS

- Chiropractic Management is provided for long-term patient care. The patients that have successfully completed their care plan and have manageable (or minimal) symptomatology are transitioned to routine chiropractic care. Patient education is the key to converting a patient from <u>active</u> treatment to <u>routine</u> chiropractic management. Any time a patient presents with unresolved or unmanageable symptoms, they are returned to an active treatment plan until improved.

BOX 5 - OPTIONS

- RED FLAG OPTIONS are available during any treatment phase. If a patient is not responding or has failed box 1 and further imaging is benign, the following is considered:
  - Order lab work for RA, SLE, HLA B27
  - Refer to a Rheumatologist
  - Refer to Family Physician or Internal Medicine Physician to check blood pressure, cardiology concerns or review lab work.

SUMMARY STATEMENT

This manual presents a foundation for designing an appropriate treatment protocol. The protocols presented are not absolutes. In designing a unique treatment protocol for individuals, there are many variables and possibilities. These proposed levels outline a methodical approach in care to eliminate failure and improve patient overall outcomes.

ADJUNCT THERAPIES

Adjunct therapies are used according to pain levels and type of pain.

- Cryo therapy (97010) is used on patients with a pain level of 5 or above. Heat should never be applied to an acute disc injury.
- Heat therapy (97010) is used for muscular restrictions or pain levels under a 5.
- Stretching therapy (97110) is performed on patients with <u>no</u> acute pain, and is avoided on patients with disc pain flared-up. Once the pain has reduced and under a 4/10, stretching is initiated as tolerated.
- Ultrasound therapy (97) is used as a tool to nourish the muscle and promote healing. Once the patient is out of the acute phase, they are transitioned to more active care than manual therapies.
- Myofascial Release / Active Release Technique (ART) (97140) can be performed every other day for muscle restrictions or nerve entrapments. Patient's muscular concerns that are not alleviated with stretching benefit greatly from myofascial treatment. It assists in lengthening the muscle that otherwise remains restricted and contracted, and assists with aligning/smoothing muscle fibers to reduce adhesions. Myofascial Release is used in conjunction with manipulation when a patient has muscle spasms in the spine region.
- Graston Technique (97110) is the use of a beveled-edge steel blade tool to assist in breaking up scar tissue or adhesions on muscle/soft tissue. When used against the grain of the adhesions, the tissue is broken down and flushed out of the body. It decreases the restriction in extension and use of the soft tissue. This cannot be performed daily, but rather every 2-3 days.
- Electrical Stimulation (G0283) is used on patients with muscular restriction as well as acute pain. Interferential methods are applied to block the pain and assist with the nerve receptors. Apply this manual therapy along with the choice of heat or cold based on patient condition.
- Cupping (97140) can be used for inflammation and restrictions. This method can be performed on patients in any pain phase. If the patient is having pain that does not decrease with conservative therapy, cupping can extract the toxins and inflammation within the muscle due to adhesions or scar tissue that otherwise remains contained in the muscle. This procedure cannot be performed daily. 2-3 days is allowed between treatments to allow the lymphatic system to flush the toxins out.
- Activator is a low-force alternative to a manual manipulation of the spine. The mechanical force manual assisted (MFMA) instrument delivers a small impulse to the spine that produces enough force to move the vertebrae and correct subluxation. If a patient is in severe pain or has a low pain threshold, the activator is a way of improving the patient experience.

COMMON PRESENTING CONDITIONS

- Neck, Back & Joint Pain
(Box 1)

- Muscle spasms/Strained Muscles
(Box 1)

- Piriformis Syndrome
(Box 1)

- Impingement Syndrome
(Box 1)

- Sprains/Strains
(Box 1)

- Scoliosis –monitor with x-rays
(Box 1)

- Disc Herniation or Bulging Disc
(Box 1/ 2 /3)

- Disc Injuries otherwise not stated
(Box 1/2/3)

- Bursitis/Tendonitis
(Box 1)

- Plantar Fascia Pain
(Box 1)

- Iliotibial Band Syndrome
(Box 1)

- Fibromyalgia
(Box 1)

- Spondylolisthesis -Grade 1
(Box 1 – with or without manipulation)

- Spondylolisthesis -Grade 2
(Box 1 –no manipulation)

- Spondylolisthesis -Grade 3
(Box 3 –no manipulation- Surgical consult immediately)

- Sciatic Nerve Pain
(Box 1/2)

- Athletic Injuries
(Box 1/2/3)

- Post-Surgical Rehab
(Box 1)

- Carpal Tunnel
(Box 1)

- TMJ Disorders
(Box 1)

- Pinched Nerves
(Box 1)

- Headaches
(Box 1)

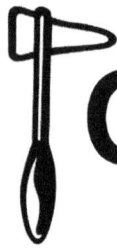

TOOL SHED &

PATIENT PROCESS

SETTING UP YOUR Tool Shed

CONSIDERATIONS FOR OFFICE SET UP

1) Aesthetic & Physical Office Environment
2) Office Policies & Procedures
3) Patient Processing & Flow
4) Electronic Medical Records

TOOL SHED SETUP & FLOW

How you set up your tool shed (aka office) can have a direct impact on your practice: its efficiency as well as the patient experience. Optimizing patient flow and efficiency are imperative to building a practice. Procedures must be smooth and consistent. Creating the right policies and procedures will produce an optimal and seamless patient flow from one treatment area to the next. Precision with procedures allows for a steady increase in patient volume and patient satisfaction.

Building your patient base begins with the patient's first moment of contact – whether it is over the telephone or in person.

Doctors must keep in mind that patients are looking for answers as well as treatment options to help alleviate their condition.

New patients are provided with a clear explanation of clinical findings, necessary referrals, treatment options, and the recommended course of treatment. For many reasons, it is important for patients to know and understand <u>why</u> they are recommended to receive specific treatments – how treatment will assist with not only alleviating symptoms but helping them achieve their health goals.

PATIENT FLOW PROCESS

Each patient is processed according to his or her needs. Patients that are scheduled as a New Patient will be processed differently than a returning patient. Similarly a patient scheduled for a diagnostic follow-up is processed differently than a patient receiving a manipulation only after their Physical Therapy.

EMR scheduling allows for appointment-types (or reason for their visit) to be assigned to each patient appointment. Therefore the staff is aware of the patients' needs, can direct the patient through the office accordingly, and can provide the doctor with the appropriate information.

Establishing consistent processes ensures more thorough evaluations and treatments, as well as timely patient appointments. Your staff additionally understands the necessities required for each patient appointment-type and can then facilitate the doctor's approach prior to seeing the patient.

INITIAL PATIENT PROCESS

CHECK IN
- All new patients check-in at front desk and complete New Patient Paperwork.
- Insurance is reviewed.
- Co-Pay and Co-Insurance information is obtained and documented.

PATIENT ROOMED
- Patient is escorted to the exam room.
- A doctor's assistant initially works-up the patient.
- Patient's history and current complaints are documented.

RADIOGRAPHIC STUDY
- With clinical indication, all new patients have imaging performed in-office for liability reasons, unless they present current imaging from a recent radiographic study.
- If a patient presents outside imaging, it is loaded and prepared for the doctor to review.
- All previous imaging reports (outside or in-office) are collected prior to doctor's initial evaluation.
- X-Rays are ordered and transferred to New Patient room. Imaging is loaded and prepared for the doctor to review during the initial evaluation.

EXAMINATION
- Doctor is then notified that the patient is ready for evaluation.
- Doctor conducts a comprehensive examination.
- Doctor reviews the radiographic study.
- Clinical findings are documented (in EMR).
- Doctor conveys to the patient the recommended treatment plan.

TREATMENT
- Treatment is rendered according to the doctor's recommended treatment plan.

REVIEW OF FINDINGS & PATIENT EDUCATION
- To avoid confusion and confirm patient understanding of the proposed course of action, the doctor's assistant reviews with the patient exam findings, treatment recommendations, referrals (if any), insurance benefits and financial obligation.
- The doctor's assistant obtains patient consent and agreement to the proposed treatment plan.
- If the patient has questions or indicates he/she cannot comply, the doctor is notified. Any and all changes or modifications requested are discussed with the doctor prior to approval and scheduling of the patient.

CHECK OUT
- All in-office appointments and referral appointments are scheduled for the patient and documented prior to their departure from the office.

NEW PATIENT PROCESS CHART

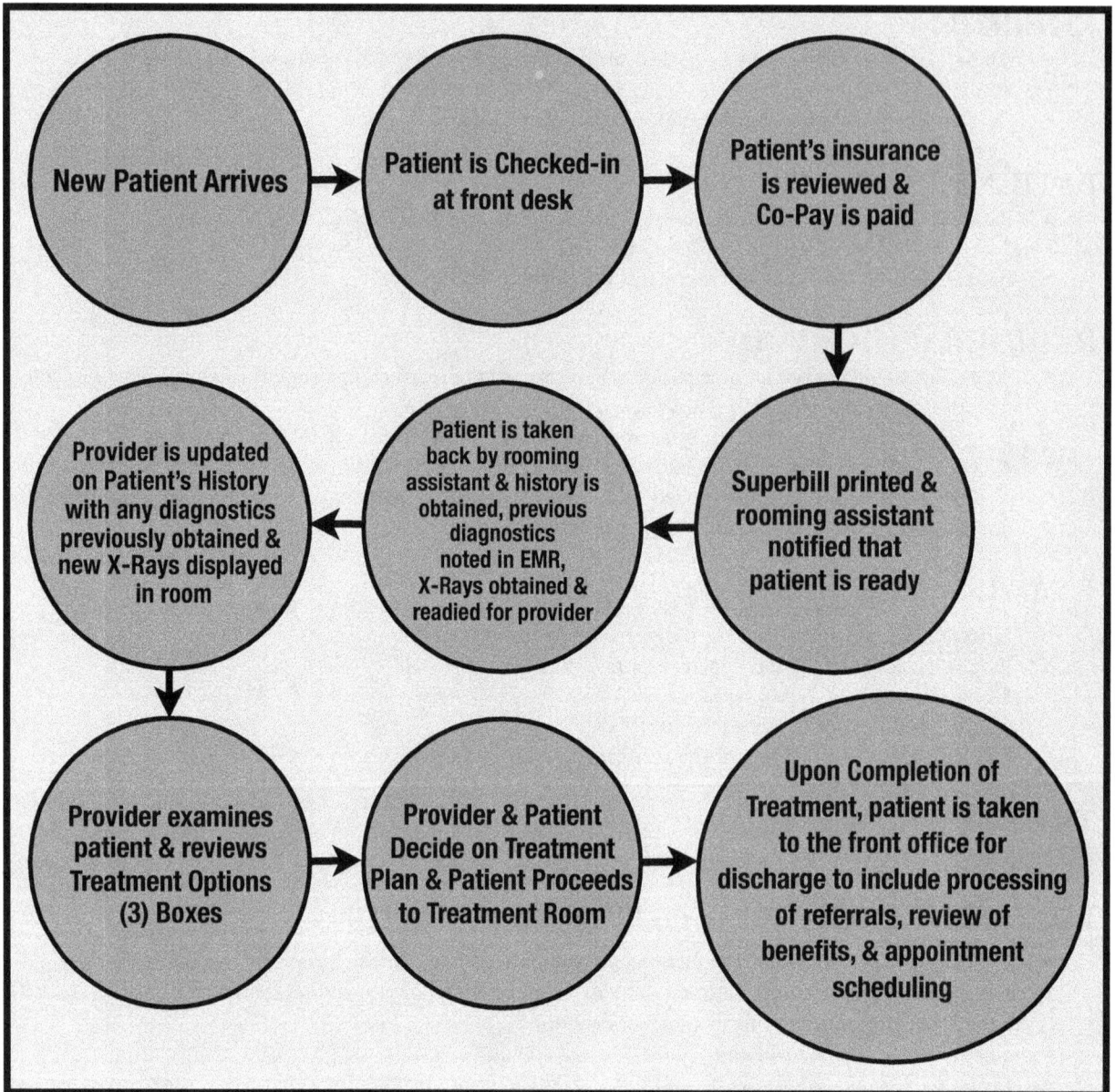

New Patient Arrives → Patient is Checked-in at front desk → Patient's insurance is reviewed & Co-Pay is paid

Provider is updated on Patient's History with any diagnostics previously obtained & new X-Rays displayed in room ← Patient is taken back by rooming assistant & history is obtained, previous diagnostics noted in EMR, X-Rays obtained & readied for provider ← Superbill printed & rooming assistant notified that patient is ready

Provider examines patient & reviews Treatment Options (3) Boxes → Provider & Patient Decide on Treatment Plan & Patient Proceeds to Treatment Room → Upon Completion of Treatment, patient is taken to the front office for discharge to include processing of referrals, review of benefits, & appointment scheduling

ESTABLISHED PATIENT PROCESS

CHECK IN

Patient arrives and checks-in at the front desk. Insurance has been obtained, verified and reviewed. Co- Pay and/or Co-Insurance is obtained. Superbill is printed and patient is placed in line to see the doctor.

PATIENT ROOMING

Patient is roomed and history is obtained and documented. Any and all diagnostics since previous visit, if current, are made available for the doctor's review.

EXAM

Doctor is updated on history. The doctor reviews diagnostics, outside referral consultations and any other patient documents. Patient is examined and findings are documented. Treatment plan is provided – if new; or continued – if existing; or modified – if improvement is noted.

TREATMENT

Patient receives manipulation if necessary. Patient is then moved to therapy area for modalities if needed. All treatment is documented.

CHECK OUT

Patient is taken to the front office. New referrals are scheduled, if recommended; new appointments are made if follow-up is needed or intra-office referrals are made. Insurance benefits are discussed if there is a change in treatment plan. All questions are answered prior to patient leaving.

ESTABLISHED PATIENT PROCESS CHART

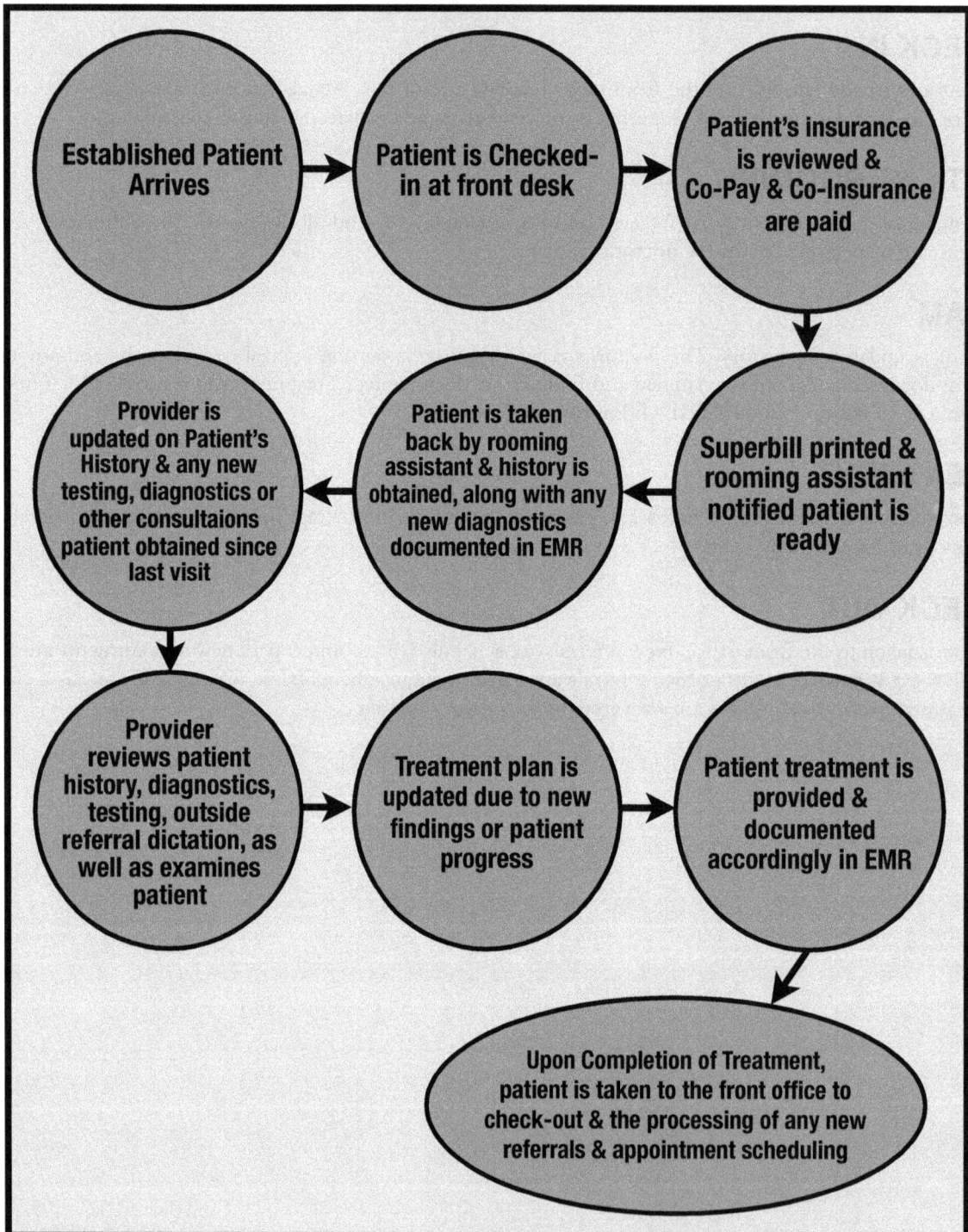

Established Patient Arrives

→

Patient is Checked-in at front desk

→

Patient's insurance is reviewed & Co-Pay & Co-Insurance are paid

↓

Superbill printed & rooming assistant notified patient is ready

←

Patient is taken back by rooming assistant & history is obtained, along with any new diagnostics documented in EMR

←

Provider is updated on Patient's History & any new testing, diagnostics or other consultaions patient obtained since last visit

↓

Provider reviews patient history, diagnostics, testing, outside referral dictation, as well as examines patient

→

Treatment plan is updated due to new findings or patient progress

→

Patient treatment is provided & documented accordingly in EMR

↓

Upon Completion of Treatment, patient is taken to the front office to check-out & the processing of any new referrals & appointment scheduling

PHYSICAL THERAPY PLUS OFFICE VISIT CHART

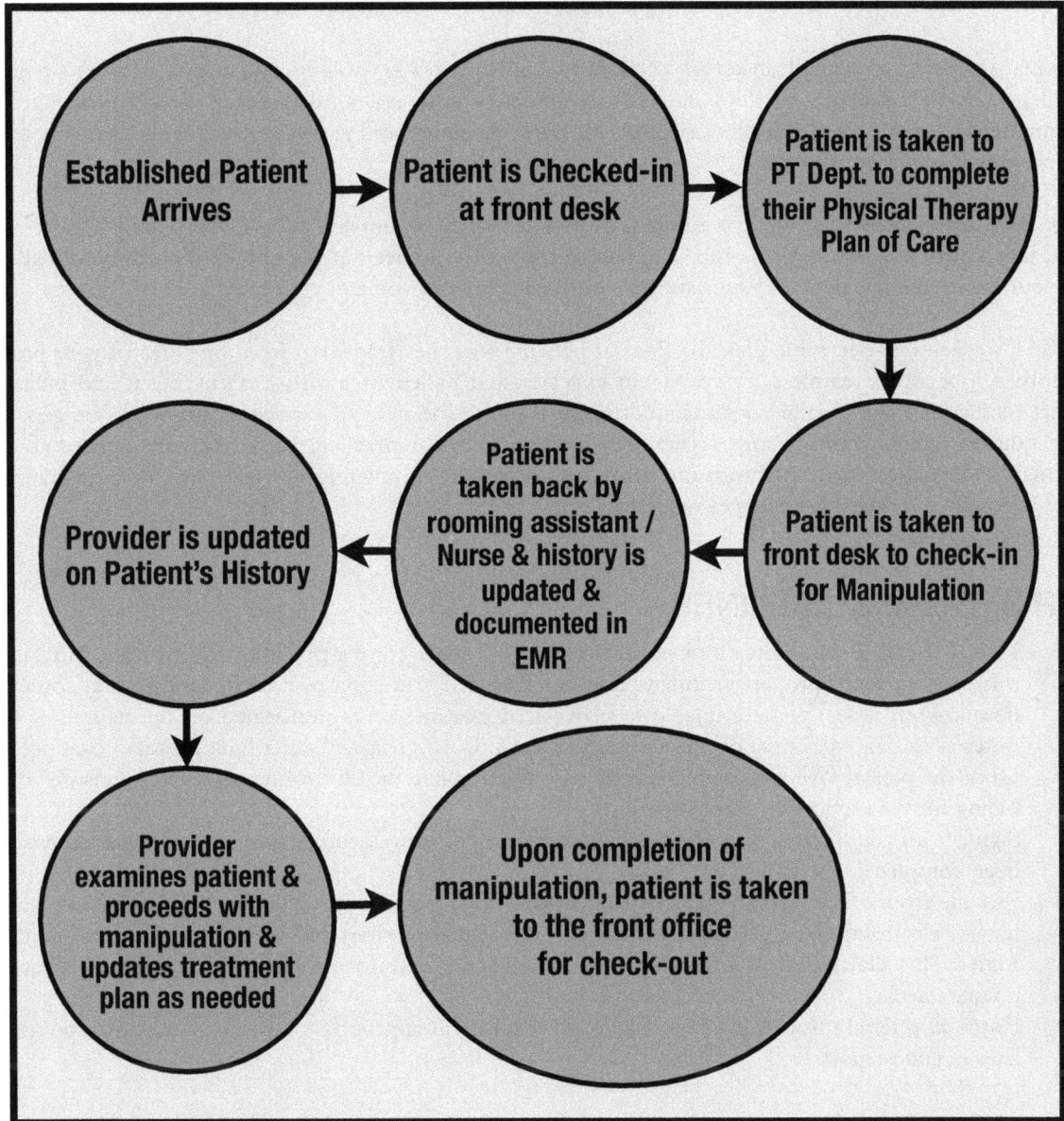

Established Patient Arrives → **Patient is Checked-in at front desk** → **Patient is taken to PT Dept. to complete their Physical Therapy Plan of Care**

Provider is updated on Patient's History ← **Patient is taken back by rooming assistant / Nurse & history is updated & documented in EMR** ← **Patient is taken to front desk to check-in for Manipulation**

Provider examines patient & proceeds with manipulation & updates treatment plan as needed → **Upon completion of manipulation, patient is taken to the front office for check-out**

OPTIMIZE EFFICIENCY WITH EMR

Electronic Medical Record (EMR) programs are now required for all healthcare systems. Although the transition from paper systems to EMR may have caused frustration and temporarily slowed down your practice (and may not seem as simple as Dictaphones and paper charting systems), they are infinitely more efficient for blending all areas of the practice and improving documentation and record retention.

Time management and immediate access to patient records plays a key role in patient care. Having a patient's complete chart (including but not limited to prior patient notes, diagnostics and outside referral documentation), readily available allows you to be more thorough and assists doctors with their decision in plan progression or modification.

Think about not having to search for a folder, or wonder where an outside referral was placed prior to being added into a patient chart. On the flip side, having the tools you need at the time you need them make not only your job easier, but elevates your patients' confidence in both you and your practice.

With easily accessible electronic files, the flow of patients – as they transition from one area of your practice to another – becomes seamless. From patient check-in and patient treatment, to check-out and billing: all aspects of the visit and care are documented in the EMR at the time of service. Reports can be generated much quicker and provide a more accurate compliance of your practice. If systems are utilized to their potential, it decreases errors of omission; it guides doctors in completing the necessary documentation to assure payment is received for services rendered.

EMR SYSTEM GUIDELINES

- Due to EMR system notes looking more uniform, never copy a previous patient note. Not only is this inaccurate for proper documentation, it's illegal. If you copy over or do not present something new in your notes, you are unable to prove that treatment was performed on the patient. Writing notes according to current events assists with tracking progress and determining patient care needs.
- Once the patient visit note is entered, be sure to complete the electronic super bill to ensure you are billing for the services you are rendering.
- Sign-off on your patient visit notes daily in order to confirm documentation for each patient visit has been completed.
- Provide front office staff all outside diagnostic information or outside doctor evaluations to scan into patient electronic chart. All files become part of a patient's chart and will be compiled in one digital folder. This allows all departments to have instant access to information needed to process a patient's unique needs.
- Enter all referral information and diagnostic requests in appropriate areas so that it may be tracked later in audit reports.

SCHEDULING & REFERRALS

APPOINTMENT SCHEDULING

Patient participation is vital. Therefore, when a patient comprehends the importance of treatment and the recommended treatment plan, they are more apt to schedule and keep appointments in compliance. Every patient has different needs and coordinating a schedule that works best with their daily activities will allow patients to adhere to the recommended treatment plan.

All referrals and treatment plans are discussed and scheduled prior to a patient leaving their initial visit. Scheduling all appointments at the start helps to gain patient commitment. It also highlights the importance of timely delivery of care and following their recommended treatment plan in order to receive the optimal outcome.

Follow-up evaluations and appointments are equally important. Patient progress determines the course of care, and the need to change and/or modify a treatment plan. Regardless of how dramatic the change may be, discussing any recommended changes in treatment with the patient provides transparency, open communication, and understanding. Every patient will progress at a different rate. Understand your options, utilize your resources, and stay current with the progress of your patients in order to modify treatment plans as necessary.

NOTE: It is important for the patient to understand the importance of their condition if left untreated. Patients that are referred for any treatment are scheduled for a follow-up appointment, with anticipation that the results from the referral appointment are promptly obtained. This promotes patient commitment and compliance.

The following are examples of scheduling for various types of treatment and follow-up.

- Patients that are referred out-of-office for imaging are scheduled for a follow up within 2 days.
- Patients referred out-of-office for physician appointments are scheduled to follow up within 1 week.
- Patients referred for Physical Therapy are scheduled within 3 days for an evaluation and a post therapy follow-up with the doctor.
- Patients referred out-of-office for lab work are scheduled for follow-up within 1 week.
- Patients recommended for injections are scheduled for the complete series of 3 injections and progress exam.

REFERRALS

Referrals are time sensitive. Whether referrals are intra-office or out-of-office, it is important to assure your referrals are processed as quickly as possible.

Establishing a trusted professional relationship with near-by specialists not only makes scheduling referral appointments succinct, it can also assist with receiving "return" referrals to your office.

Using a comprehensive Referral Form provides detailed information to the referral specialist to assist with gathering the necessary clinical information. Any patient information obtained in-office related to the referral appointment is forwarded with the Referral Request to expedite the appointment. Without the proper documentation, the referral doctor resorts to guesswork. Often times when a referral doctor is unclear of the purpose it complicates the appointment, and their evaluation can yield confusing diagnosis' that ultimately do not provide clarity for your recommended treatment plan. Unclear communication to the referral doctor also clouds patient expectation and decreases patient confidence in your clinical competency.

Follow-up is mandatory. Without this procedure, referrals slip through the cracks and can delay the treatment process for a patient. Again, all referrals and treatment plans are discussed and scheduled prior to a patient leaving for their referral appointment. If not promptly scheduled, the referral then appears to be more of a recommendation than a necessity. When a patient understands the purpose of the referral, the plan of care (including the importance of gathering information through additional diagnostic studies), they are more compliant with following doctor recommendations.

Type of Referral	Scheduled Next Visit	Type of Visit
Out-of-office Radiographic Referral	within 2 days	Follow-up
Out-of-office Physician/Specialist Referral	within 1 week	Follow-up
Intra-office Physical Therapy	within 3 days	Evaluation & Follow-up
Out-of-office Lab Work	within 1 week	Follow-up & Lab Review
Intra-office Injections	after 3 injections	Progress Exam

PHYSICIAN ORDERS EXAMPLE

REFERRAL ORDERS

Patient Name:_____   Date: _____

Dr. _____

_____   **STAT**

_____   **MRI**   C _____   T _____   L _____   Follow-up Date: _____
           Date Scheduled: _____

_____   **Chiropractic**
                     DAILY / ____ Days x ___ Weeks   Chiro Only / Chiro + Physical Medicine

_____   **Physical Therapy**
           First Evaluation: _____   PT Only / PT + Manipulation

_____   **Pain Management**
           Referred to Dr. _____

                _____   **Medication**   Steroid Pack / Muscle Relaxers / Other: _____
                _____   **Injection**

           Type   ESI   FACET   SNRB   Other: _____
                         Level: _____
                         R   L   Bilateral

_____   **Neurological Consult**
           Referred to Dr. _____   Follow-up Date: _____

_____   **Neurosurgeon**
           Referred to Dr. _____   Follow-up Date: _____

_____   **Orthopedic Surgeon**
           Referred to Dr. _____   Follow-up Date: _____

_____   **Other**

           _____
           _____

Notes:

_____
_____
_____

EXAMPLE NOTES

Visit Note

Provider

Supervising: Doctor Name
Performing: Doctor Name

Encounter Date: Jan 01, 2015

Patient: Test, Austina A (PT00000010)
Gender: Female
DOB: Jun 06, 1970 Age: 44 year
Address: 123 XYZ Street, Austin TX 73301
Insurance: BLUE CROSS BLUE SHIELD

Chief Complaint

Ms. Test is a 43 year old female who presents to the office for treatment. Ms. Test has a history of cervical and thoracic pain. She has chosen to treat her condition conservatively. This patient is having a reoccurrence of neck and mid back symptoms. She contributes her current symptoms to her job as a computer data analyst. She has had an increase in overtime at work. Patient describes her symptoms as achy, dull and tight. She is not experiencing radiating pain as a result of her symptoms. She reports not having any new injuries since her last visit. Ms. Test is here today requesting an adjustment. She has stated her pain level is a 3 /10 She has not taken any medications for her symptoms. She has not had any diagnostic testing or outside consultations since her last visit.

ROS

Genitourinary: Patient does not report change in bladder complaints, urinary incontinence, blood or burning on urination, unless otherwise noted.

Neurological: Current findings are noted below. Additional findings may be noted in the initial history.

Psychological: Patient does not report change in history of depression or other disorders, unless otherwise noted herein.

ENT: Patient does not report change in equilibrium or other symptoms unless otherwise noted.

Endocrinological: Patient does not report change in abnormal fatigue or other endocrinological problems, unless otherwise noted.

Dermatological: Patient does not report change in or complaints of rashes, hives or any other dermatological pathology, unless otherwise noted.

Cardiovascular: Patient does not report change in or development of shortness of breath, positional hypotension, hypertension, dizziness or any other problems unless otherwise noted.

Pulmonary: Patient does not report change in or development of pulmonary edema or related type of symptoms, unless otherwise noted.

Musculoskeletal: As seen in the nature of presenting problems and explained herein, unless otherwise noted.

Physical Examination

Point Tenderness/ Restrictions:

Patient has maximum point tenderness upon palpation bilaterally in the cervical paraspinal muscle. There bilateral cervical rotation; C-4 to 6; T-3, T-4 restrictions.

Alignment/ Postural:

There are cervical and thoracic end point facet restrictions. Examination shows straightening of the cervical spine with moderate loss of the normal cervical lordosis. Patient has postural changes as indicated: forward head posture forward rolled shoulders.

ROM of Regions:

Patient presents pain with cervical extension. Patient does not appear to have pain with cervical flexion. Patient has decreased joint motion. Patient has 75% of normal cervical range of motion.

Tissue/ Muscle Tightness

Patient has abnormal tissue/muscle hypertonicity bilaterally in the cervical spinalis muscle and bilateral upper trapezius muscle.

Orthopedic/Neuro Testing

Orthopedic examination reveals the following findings: Premanipulative testing is negative.
Neuro examination reveals normal sensory findings.

Cervical Spine Orthopedic Tests

(-) Jackson Compression Test.
(-) Shoulder Depression Test.

Diagnosis:

722.4 Cervical Disc Degeneration
723.4 Cervical Radiculitis
724.1 Thoracic Pain

Daily Patient Therapy Note

Ms. Test was treated, as requested by the performing provider, with 1 unit of electrical stimulation, 1 unit of manual therapy and a hot/cold pack. The following modalities were performed by: Chiro technician #2.

Pre-Pain Level 3 Post-Pain level 1 Time therapy started: 12.15 Time therapy stopped: 1.10.

Treatment was performed to her cervical region. Ice was applied to the patient due to her current symptoms. The patient stated they felt improved and decreased muscle tightness following her treatment today.

Stretching

Cervical Stretching: Neck Rotation Neck Flexion Neck Extension Levator Scapula Stretch.

Plan

Individual / Additional Adjustment:
The patient was treated with manipulation to the Cervical and Thoracic region.
Modalities were provided and patient reported relief.
Ms. Test was explained the treatment and received the same with no complications. The patient has no further questions at this time.

Goals

Short Term: decrease pain; increase range of motion.

Visit Frequency/ Follow-up

Patient will be treated three times a week and re-evaluated after that time.

EXAMPLE NOTES 2

Visit Note

Provider
Supervising: Dr. Supervising
Performing: Dr. Performing

Encounter Date: Jan 02, 2015

Patient: Tester, Austina A (PT00000020)
Gender: Female DOB: Jun 06, 1971 Age: 43 year
Address: 123 XYZ Street, Austin TX 73301
Insurance: BLUE CROSS BLUE SHIELD

New Patient

New Patient Intake
Patient presents to the office today with neck and lower back pain. She began feeling a tight sensation 2 weeks ago over the holidays while on a 14-hour road trip. Her pain appears to be worsening. She has had chronic cervical and lumbar pain, but has been able to resolve her symptoms in the past, OTC medication and rest. Since her recent flare up, the patient is experiencing numbness in her arms and hands as well as a tingling sensation in her leg. Her back starts hurting if she sits for any extended period of time. She stated she is unable to sleep at night without waking up with pain in her neck and low back. She has been trying OTC medication again and has not felt improvement.

Pain Level (__ /10): On a scale of 1 to 10, ten being the worst pain imaginable, the patient rated her pain as 7.

Factors that Improve pain: She does not feel the increased intensity of pain while using heat.

Factors that make pain worse: She feels worse with laying down, sitting, walking and lifting.

Have you been treated previously?: Yes. The patient has not tried any kind of treatment for her problem. The patient has not had any diagnostic test performed.

Height (Feet. Inches): 5.4.   **Weight** (lbs): 160.

Review of Systems
Gastrointestinal: No history of ulcers, diarrhea, constipation or other gastrointestinal complaints, other than noted in the initial history.
Genitourinary: No bladder complaints, urinary incontinence, retention, blood or burning on urination, other than noted in initial history.
Neurological: has bilateral cervical radiculopathy with paresthesias; no weakness or abnormalities of gait, proprioception, memory loss, or confusion, other than noted in the initial history.
Psychological: No history of depression, neurotic or psychotic disorders, other than noted in the initial history.
ENT: No complaints of loss of equilibrium or other ENT problems, other than if noted in the initial history.
Endocrinological: No complaints relative to temperature insensitivity or hypersensitivity, abnormal fatigue, diabetes, thyroid dysfunction, or other endocrinological problems, other than noted in the initial history.
Dermatological: No complaints of rashes, hives or lesions, no history of maculae, papules or any other dermatological pathology, other than noted in the initial history.

Cardiovascular: No shortness of breath, positional hypotension, history of hypertension, dizziness, transient ischemic attacks or any other problems, other than noted in the initial history.

Family History

The patient's family history is noncontributory.

Medical History

All past medical history was reviewed. There is no previous history of the same or similar condition. No known drug allergies. No serious illnesses or surgeries. Patient does not have a history of cancer. Patient does not have a history of diabetes. Patient does not have a history of heart disease.
Patient does have a history of high blood pressure. Patient has not been checked for Rheumatoid / Lupus. Patient does not have a history of thyroid problems

Social History

The patient does not smoke; does drink; exercises frequently.

Physical Examination

X-Rays were performed and reviewed. Findings appear to have questions and will therefore be sent for a Radiology review.

General: Observation of the patient's general appearance revealed a person who is well developed, of adequate nutrition, seems to be well groomed and maintained, and without any deformities unless noted below.

Musculoskeletal: The patient's gait and station were normal. An assessment was made of motor function. Upper extremity strength was normal. Lower extremity strength was normal. There was no noted muscle atrophy or movements unless noted below.

Neurological: Testing is found to be normal unless noted in pertinent exam below. The patient was well oriented to time, space and person. Recent and remote memory appeared to be intact. The patient's attention span and memory appeared to be normal. There did not appear to be any difficulty with language or general awareness. There appears to be S1 dysthesias. Deep tendon reflexes were tested and found to be within normal limits. Coordination testing was negative.

Pertinent Exam

Point Tenderness/ Restrictions:

Patient has maximum point cervical tenderness and guarding. There are bilateral cervical rotation restrictions, T5-9 thoracic and L4 to S1 lumbar restrictions.

Alignment/ Postural:

There are cervical, thoracic and lumbar end point facet restrictions. Examination shows straightening of the cervical spine with loss of the normal cervical lordosis. Patient has postural changes as indicated: forward head posture, forward rolled shoulders. Patient has a left lumbar deviation in spine.

ROM of Regions:

Patient presents pain with cervical and lumbar extension, cervical flexion and bilateral cervical rotation.

Tissue/ Muscle Tightness:

Patient has abnormal tissue/muscle hypertonicity in the right lumbar erector spinea muscles.

Patient is experiencing bilateral sternocleidomastoideus and bilateral trapezius muscle spasms.

Orthopedic/Neuro Examination:

Orthopedic examination reveals the following findings: Premanipulative testing is negative.

Cervical Spine Orthopedic Tests

(+) Foraminal Compression Test (bilateral). (+) Shoulder Depression Test.

Lumbar Spine Orthopedic Tests:

(-) Heel/Toe Walk Test. The patient does not have any weakness during heel/toe walk.

(+) Kemp Test. Compression causes or aggravates the pattern of radicular pain that is suggestive of nerve root compression.

(-) Minor Sign. The patient is not trying to support weight on the uninvolved side.

(+) Straight-Leg-Raise Test. right sided back pain only Symptomatology was elicited with flexion of the thigh on the pelvis and flexion of the lumbar spine which is suggestive of lumbosacral or sacroiliac lesions, disc lesions, spondylolisthesis, adhesions, or intervertebral foramen occlusion. Patient has pain that radiates thru the shoulders bilaterally and down into the hands and last 2 digits of each hand.

Neurologic Exam

Patient has bilateral arm and hand and right leg paresthesias.

X-Ray Findings: X-Ray Findings are as follows: Cervical: loss of lordosis, decreased disc space at C5/6 and C6/7, moderate anterior osteophytes at C4, C5 & C6. Lumbar: left deviation, decreased disc space at L5/S1 with a transitional vertebra at S1.

Diagnosis

722.4 Cervical Disc Degeneration   723.4 Cervical Radiculitis   722.52 Lumbar Disc Degeneration
724.4 Lumbar Radiculitis

Plan

Patient's plan will be modified as follows:

Treatment Referrals: MRI Study: Patient will be referred for a Cervical and Lumbar MRI to rule out more serious pathology based on objective findings and will be reviewed upon their follow up visit.

Physician Referrals

Ms. Test will be referred to Dr. Feelbetter for a pain management for a consultation.

The patient has been referred to their family physician or closest emergency facility to rule out any non-musculoskeletal reasons for their symptoms or if symptomatology increases.

I have discussed treatment with the patient. No guarantees were given, neither expressed nor implied, and informed consent was obtained.

Treatment option chosen: Patient was informed of the rehabilitative spine guidelines we follow. These three levels of treatment options being conservative care including physical therapy and chiropractic management, traction with or without injections and our last resort of surgery. Patient has chosen conservative care pending her MRIs.

Complete Adjustment

The patient was treated with manipulation to the cervical, thoracic and lumbar spine region.

Ms. Test was explained the treatment and received the same with no complications. The patient has no further questions at this time.

Goals

Short Term: decrease pain; increase range of motion.

Visit Frequency/ Follow-up

Patient will be treated daily this week with modalities, manipulation if necessary, and re-evaluated after that time.

Diagnostic/Lab
Point Diagnostics:
MRI- CERVICAL SPINE NON-CONTRAST.
MRI - LUMBAR SPINE NON-CONTRAST

Note Dictation Templates

Let's face it, documenting patient exams and treatments can break or make your practice. If not done properly, you become vulnerable to authorities, can mis-direct patients, and have poor out-comes. However, when you have a solid system in place and document appropriately, it creates clarity for anyone requesting copies of patient files, promotes quality patient care, and nurtures successful outcomes.

Below are examples of detailed templates created by Dr. Akerman to thoroughly explain the service(s) rendered:

- **CERVICAL STRETCHING –** The patient was shown the cervical stretching protocol including flexion, extension, rotation, lateral flexion (bilateral), and chin tucks using eccentric loading. The patient was shown exercises in great detail and given exact duration and frequency. Patient was given handout with detailed description of activities and directions for activity completion.

- **CERVICAL ISOMETRIC PROTOCOL – The** patient was shown the cervical isometric protocol including flexion, extension, lat flexion, rotation, retraction, and protraction for intrinsic muscles of the cervical spine using isometric contractions. The patient was shown exercises in great detail and given exact duration and frequency. Patient was given handout with detailed description of activities and directions for activity completion.

- **CERVICAL ISOTONIC PROTOCOL –** The patient was shown the cervical isotonic protocol including flexion, extension, lat flexion, rotation, retraction, protraction for intrinsic muscles of the cervical spine using isotonic contractions with a soft ball and a wall. The patient was shown exercises in great detail and given exact duration and frequency. Patient was given handout with detailed description of activities and directions for activity completion.

- **CERVICAL POSTURAL EXERCISES –** The patient was shown postural exercises including isometric contraction of extrinsic muscles of the cervical and mid-thoracic spine including scapular retraction. The patient was shown exercises in great detail and given exact duration and frequency. Patient was given handout with detailed description of activities and directions for activity completion.

- **THORACIC POSTURAL PROTOCOL –** The patient was shown the thoracic postural protocol including latissimus dorsi and rhomboids isokinetic exercises using a Thera-Band. The patient was shown exercises in great detail and given exact duration and frequency. Patient was given handout with detailed description of activities and directions for activity completion.

- **LUMBAR STRETCHING PROTOCOL –** The patient was shown the lumbar stretching protocol including knee to chest, double knee to chest, piriformis, hamstring, calf, and pelvic tilt using eccentric loading. The patient was shown exercises in great detail and given exact duration and frequency. Patient was given handout with detailed description of activities and directions for activity completion.

- **LUMBAR STRENGTHENING PROTOCOL-1 –** The patient was shown lumbar strengthening protocol 1 including paraspinal erector spinal, straight leg raise, double leg raise using isotonic contractions. The patient was shown exercises in great detail and given exact duration and frequency. Patient was given handout with detailed description of activities and directions for activity completion.

- **LUMBAR STRENGTHENING PROTOCOL-2 –** The patient was shown lumbar strengthening protocol 2 including bridging, cross crawl, planks. The patient was shown exercises in great detail and given exact duration and frequency. Patient was given handout with detailed description of activities and directions for activity completion.

- **LUMBAR STRENGTHENING PROTOCOL-3 –** The patient was shown lumbar strengthening protocol 3 including bridging, cross crawl, planks, leg raises using a Swiss ball. The patient was shown exercises in great detail and given exact duration and frequency. Patient was given handout with detailed description of activities and directions for activity completion.

ADMINISTRATIVE

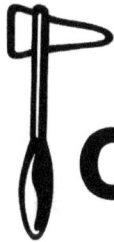

Tools FOR

FINANCIAL SUCCESS

COLLECTING MONEY FOR THE USE OF YOUR TOOLS

ADMINISTRATIVE TOOLS

The ability to bill and collect for your services is an area that is seldom discussed in school and is one of, if not the most important asset to the tool shed aka: your practice. Over the course of 18+ years of practice this area has remained consistently difficult to manage, as the rules and documentation requirements are ever changing. The days when a doctor could simply treat a patient, bill the service and be paid are a fading memory.

Today doctor's must diagnose, treat, pre-authorize, document, bill, and then start the collection process – and pray for the best. The future is all about documentation as we see the implementation of ICD-10 in the near future. 2014 introduces the first wave of government-backed health care plans. With lots of 'unknowns' it will probably become more difficult before any reprieve.

This being said, you need to have a thorough understanding of the billing process. Would it surprise you to know billing begins at patient intake? The importance of 'getting it right' and assuring your patients understand their responsibility are not only vital to your reputation but also your pocketbook. As mentioned, the day and age of doing a service and simply getting paid are long gone. This chapter walks you through the process and identifies the resources needed to assure you collect for using any of the tools in our tool shed.

PATIENT INTAKE PROCESS FOR FINANCIAL SUCCESS

Patient Intake can also break or make any practice; this is where you must get it right. If you are not a cash based practice, who is going to pay you for the services you deliver? It sounds like a simple question, but as the insurance carriers have continued to change and modify benefits this becomes a crucial area in any practice. It has to be right from the beginning.

Over the years we have developed and re-developed the forms we use on a daily basis. We have designed payer type explicit forms to address the information necessary to process claims. The Patient Intake Process our practice established assures payment for services rendered and your patient's clear understanding of their financial responsibility.

PATIENT INTAKE PROCESS

Step 1 - Patient Calls in inquiring about your services and wanting to make an appointment.

Step 2 – Staff determines the type of patient.

Step 3 - Staff Completes the appropriate Insurance Verification Form for Benefit Processing.
   A. Group Insurance Payer Form, i.e.: BCBS, Aetna, Cigna, United Health Care, Medicare, etc.
   B. Workers Compensation Form - This form is used for injured workers.
   C. Auto Accident Form - This form is used for any person using Personal Injury Protection or a Letter of Protection from an Attorney.

Step 4 - Appointment is scheduled.

Step 5 - Staff calls and verifies data collected with insurance carriers.
   A. Obtains referral from Primary Care Provider if required with an HMO policy.
   B. Verifies Workers Compensation claim.
   C. Obtains a Letter of Protection for Attorney cases.

Step 6 - Benefits are loaded into Practice Management Software (EMR).

Step 7 - Staff calls patient to review benefits/case status and explain patient responsibility.

We have found that step seven is critical to getting the patient established with a complete understanding of their benefits and their financial responsibility. Over the years we have found that most patients do not understand their benefits. They tend to believe their co-payment covers everything. The truth is, it usually only covers the office visit. Making sure your patient understands their benefits is critical. It has to be right from the beginning.

PATIENT INTAKE CHART

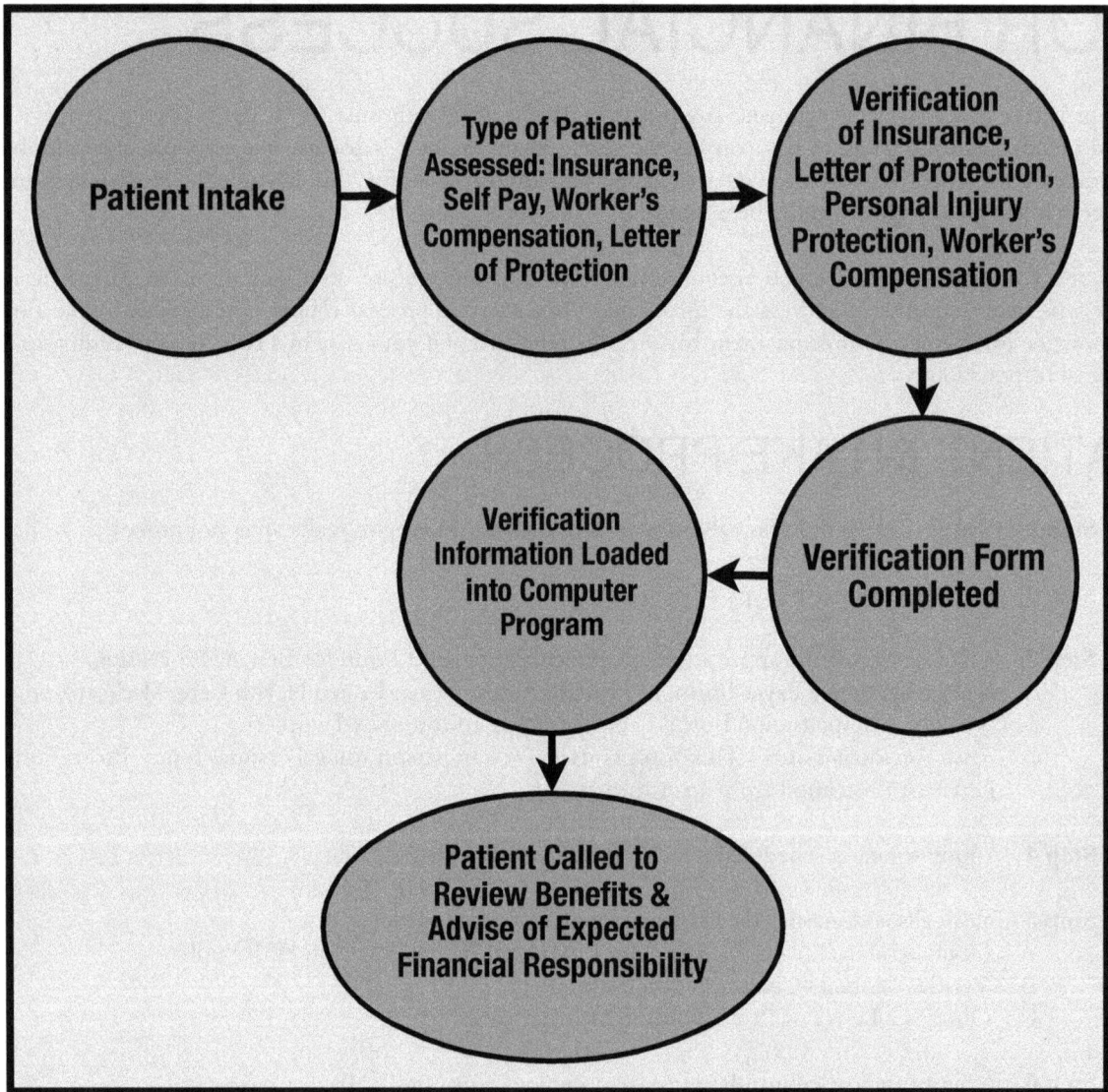

Patient Intake

Type of Patient Assessed: Insurance, Self Pay, Worker's Compensation, Letter of Protection

Verification of Insurance, Letter of Protection, Personal Injury Protection, Worker's Compensation

Verification Information Loaded into Computer Program

Verification Form Completed

Patient Called to Review Benefits & Advise of Expected Financial Responsibility

MARK YEZAK B.S., D.C.

INSURANCE VERIFICATION FORM

Patient Name: _____ DOB: _____ Phone: _____

Address:_____ Apt #:_____ Secondary Phone: _____

Referred By: _____ Email: _____

Parent / Spouse Name: _____ Complaint(s): _____

_____

Diagnostic: ( ) Yes ( ) No   Date of Study: _____   Type(s): _____ Body Region(s): _____

INSURANCE INFORMATION: SUBSCRIBER NAME: _____ EMPLOYER: _____

Insurance Company: _____   HMO/PPO:_____ Phone: _____

TO WHO ARE CLAIMS MAILED? Claims Address: _____ Payer ID: _____

Patient ID: _____   Group #: _____   Effective Date: _____   Calendar YR or Benefit PD

Referral Needed: ( ) Yes ( ) No PCP Name: _____   Phone: _____

H.S.A./H.R.A. ( ) Yes ( ) No

BEGINNING AMOUNT: _____   **ACCT BALANCE:**_____   **PATIENT** OR **EMPLOYER MANAGED (circle one)**

Doctor NPI _____   **TIN #** _____   **PRACTICE NPI** _____   **TIN #**_____

PHYSICAL THERAPY BENEFITS (OFFICE SETTING):

Ded $ _____   Ded met $ _____   Fam Ded $ _____   Fam Ded Met $ _____

Co-Pay $ _____   Coins: _____/_____   *Note: _____

OOP $ _____   OOP met $ _____   Fam OOP $ _____   Fam OOP Met $ _____

Circle all that apply: CP DED COINS apply to OOP.   In-Network to Out-Of-Network Cross Accumulation? ( ) Yes ( ) No

Visit Max #/$ _____   Pre-Auth Required: ( ) **Yes** ( ) **No**   Is Visit Max a Hard Max? ( ) **Yes** ( ) **No**

Will the PT visits accumulate toward the visit max **DURING** or **AFTER** the deductible is met?

Massage Therapy: ( ) **Yes** ( ) **No**   DME (E0730-TENS unit): ( ) **Yes** ( ) **No**   In-Network Benefit: _____

MEDICAL SPEC OV:

Doctor NPI _____   **TIN #** _____   **PRACTICE NPI** _____   **TIN #** _____

Ded $ _____   Ded met $ _____   Fam Ded $ _____   Fam Ded Met $ _____

Co-Pay $ _____   Coins: _____/_____   *Note: _____

OOP $ _____   OOP met $ _____   Fam OOP $ _____   Fam OOP Met $ _____

* Are X-rays inclusive in office visit? ( ) **Yes** ( ) **No** / If not included what co-insurance/co-pay is applicable?_____
* If a patient receives therapy services during an office visit, are the therapy services inclusive with the OV co-pay or does co-insurance apply in addition to the OV co-pay? ( ) **Yes** ( ) **No**
* Is pre-cert required for following CPT codes: ( ) **64483** ( ) **64484** ( ) **64490** ( ) **64491** ( ) **20610** ( ) **62311**

OUT OF NETWORK:

Ded $ _____   Ded met $ _____   Fam Ded $ _____   Fam Ded Met $ _____

Co-Pay $ _____   Coins: _____/_____   *Note: _____

OOP $ _____   OOP met $ _____   Fam OOP $ _____   Fam OOP Met $ _____

Whom spoken to/Reference #: _____Verified By: _____ Date: _____NPT_____

ADMINISTRATIVE TOOLS FOR FINANCIAL SUCCESS

WORK COMP INSURANCE INTAKE FORM

PATIENT NAME: _____ EMAIL: _____

SSN: _____ DOB: _____

ADDRESS:
_____

PHONE: (CELL) _____ (HOME) _____

EMPLOYER NAME: _____ PHONE: _____

ADDRESS: _____ FAX (FOR 73): _____

DOI: _____ TIME OF INJURY: _____ SHIFT BEGIN/END: _____ DATE REPORTED: _____

COMPLAINTS:
_____

INITIAL CALL QUESTIONNAIRE

HOW DID THE INJURY OCCUR? _____

_____

DID YOU VISIT AN ER?   Y or N   EMS TRANSPORT? Y or N   DATE VISITED ER: _____ ER NAME: _____
(MEDICATIONS/DIAGNOSTICS/WORK STATUS/FOLLOW UP W/ CO. DOCTOR):

_____

_____

DISPUTED: ( ) Y ( ) N   IN NETWORK CLAIM: ( ) Y ( ) N   DR. THAI IN NETWORK: ( ) Y ( ) N   TXID: 47-0862283

INSURANCE COMPANY: _____ EMPLOYER/CLAIM NETWORK:_____

ADDRESS: _____ INSURANCE CO. PHONE: _____

ADJUSTER: _____ PHONE: _____

ADJUSTER EMAIL: _____ FAX : _____

CLAIM NUMBER: _____ COMPENSABLE INJURY: _____

PRE-AUTHORIZATION COMPANY: _____ PRE-AUTH PHONE: _____

PRE-AUTH FAX: _____

REFERRING DOCTOR: _____ REFERRING DOCTOR PHONE: _____

REFERRING DOCTOR FAX: _____ TREATING DOCTOR: _____

TREATING DOCTOR PHONE: _____ TREATING DOCTOR FAX: _____

PT FACILITIES IN NETWORK: RSA TXID: 26-4473117   ( ) Y ( ) N   HSRC TXID: 76-0594342   ( ) Y ( ) N

INS. CO. REPRESENTATIVE NAME: _____ VERIFIED BY: _____ DATE: _____

MARK YEZAK B.S., D.C.

AUTO ACCIDENT INSURANCE VERIFICATION

Patient Name: _____ DOB: _____ Phone: _____

Address: _____ Email: _____

Referred By: _____ SS#: _____

Diagnostic: **Y** or **N**   Date of Study: _____ Type(s): _____ Body Region(s): _____

Date of Injury: _____ ER Name: _____ EMS: **Y** or **N**

Complaints Resulting from Accident:_____

Is Patient Currently Being Treated for Pre-existing Injuries? Y or N Injuries: _____

_____

ATTORNEY INFORMATION:

Attorney/Firm Name: _____   Phone: _____

Address: _____   Fax: _____

Case Manager: _____   Email: _____

DETAILS OF THE ACCIDENT:

Other passengers? **Y** or **N** Name(s): _____Injuries: _____

Police Report Filed? **Y** or **N**   Is Vehicle Drivable? **Y** or **N**   Did You Have Pictures of Damages?   **Y** or **N**

Damage To Vehicle: _____ Own or Lease? _____ Rental on Policy? **Y** or **N**

1.)   PATIENT'S AUTO INSURANCE INFORMATION:

Insurance Company: _____   Phone: _____

Claims Mailing Address: _____

Policy #: _____ Claim #: _____ PIP Coverage Amount: _____

Adjuster Name: _____ Fax #: _____ □ Proof of Declination □ Declined Coverage

2.)   PATIENT'S HEALTH INSURANCE INFORMATION:

Insurance Company: _____ HMO/PPO: _____ Phone: _____

Claims Mailing Address: _____

Circle One:

Patient ID: _____ Group #: _____ Effective Date: _____ Calendar YR or Benefit PD

Referral Needed: Y or N   PCP Name: _____ Phone: _____

Representative/Reference#: (1)_____ (2)_____ Verified By: _____ Date: _____

REFERRAL RECEIVED _____   EMAILED _____   NPT ENTERED _____

VERIFIED INSURANCE EXPLANATION - FOR PATIENT

Patient Benefits and Patient Responsibility Acknowledgement

Dear _____,   Date: _____

The _____ insurance information you have provided was verified on_____.

The following is a breakdown of your insurance benefits and expected financial responsibility for your office visit and any therapy services provided during that visit.

Your Specialist Office Visit and Therapy Benefits:

When you see a doctor in our office, the office visit is covered: _____.

When you have therapies in the office, the services are covered: _____.

You are allowed _____ visits of therapy/PT.

_____ are services that are not covered by your insurance carrier & the patient responsibility per date of service will be: _____.

Your Deductible is $ _____ and has been / not been satisfied.

Your remaining deductible is $ _____.

You do / do not have an HSA or HRA account. Balance of HSA/HRA is: $ _____ .

Prescription of Care:

Dr. _____ has prescribed: _____

_____

Expected Patient Responsibility Per Date of Service:

For your prescribed plan of care, your expected estimated patient responsibility per date of service is:

Visits _____ through _____ the estimated daily patient responsibility will be: _____.

Visits _____ through _____ the estimated daily patient responsibility will be: _____.

Visits _____ through _____ the estimated daily patient responsibility will be: _____.

Plan of Care Re-evaluation Date and Benefit Re-evaluation Date: _____.
_____

I understand total charges for services provided are my responsibility less any amounts paid by my insurance carrier as well as any contractual adjustments from my carrier. I also understand that depending on my response to the prescription of care, that the doctor may amend the treatment plan to better benefit my condition.

Printed Name:_____

Patient Signature:_____ Date:_____

*Co-Insurance for therapy services may not be collected with the office visit Co-Pay or Co-Insurance but will be billed to the patient once insurance payment is received.
*Co-Insurance for office visit will be collected at the time of service and will be based on an average visit of $100. This amount should average out in the course of treatment but once insurance payment is received patient will be responsible for any remaining Co-Insurance.

ASSURING FINANCIAL SUCCESS THROUGH VISIT PROCESS

After the intake, the visit process is up to the practitioners. The step-by-step process a patient moves through not only sets the foundation for their first impression of your practice but it sets the tone for how your patient feels about their experience, your practice and coming to you for care. Practice procedures are an ever-changing area of any practice, however they are also one of the most important areas. It truly starts from the very beginning.

The following procedures work to assure your patient understands their treatment plan and financial responsibility with receiving care in your office.

VISIT PROCESS OVERVIEW

Patient is WELCOMED to the practice with a BRIGHT greeting.

> Why is that Important?
> First impressions are **EVERYTHING!**

Then, the patient INTAKE:

- Name Verified
- Address Change Noted
- Co-Payment/ Co-Insurance Collected
  - o If Patient has a balance, make every effort to collect the amount due in order to reduce billing costs and post service effort.
- Patient is then invited to begin the Office Visit
  - o Patient is assessed and work-up performed and documented accordingly.
  - o Practitioner then evaluates, diagnoses, and provides treatment plan and documents.
  - o Super bill completed to include diagnosis and level of office service and therapy services provided.
- Visit Completion Process
  - o Treatment plan is reviewed; scheduling is performed.
  - o Financial expectations are explained and issues addressed.
  - o Referrals are managed and scheduled:
    - Send outside referrals i.e. MRI, Outside Providers, Physical Therapy, Lab, etc.
    - Pre-Authorization for treatment prescribed in treatment plan, if required
  - o Address any scheduling issues or concerns and adjust plan to meet your Patient's needs.

REMEMBER IT IS YOUR REPUTATION.
MAKE CUSTOMER SERVICE YOUR PRACTICE PLATFORM.

VISIT PROCESS CHART

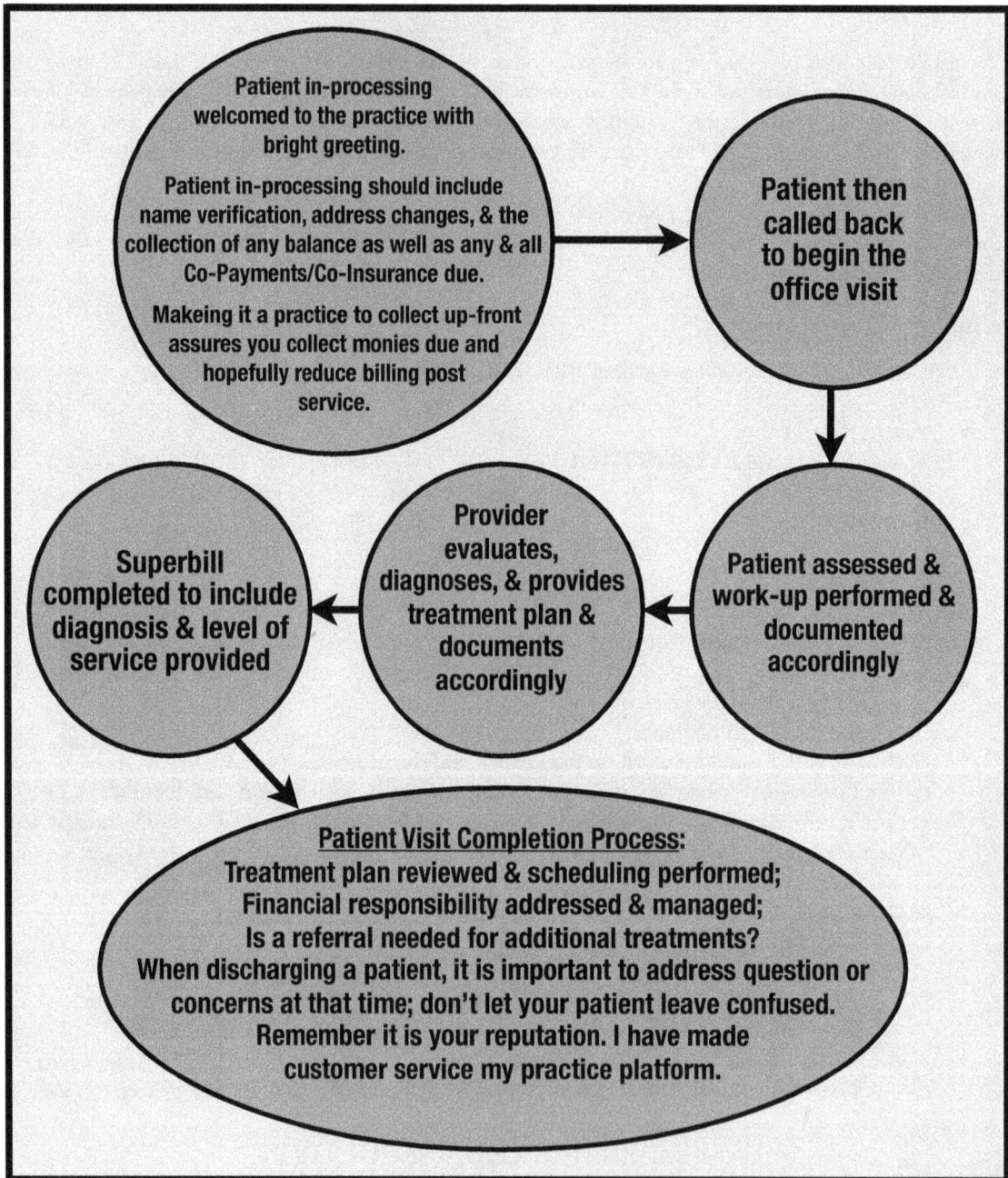

Patient in-processing welcomed to the practice with bright greeting.

Patient in-processing should include name verification, address changes, & the collection of any balance as well as any & all Co-Payments/Co-Insurance due.

Makeing it a practice to collect up-front assures you collect monies due and hopefully reduce billing post service.

Patient then called back to begin the office visit

Patient assessed & work-up performed & documented accordingly

Provider evaluates, diagnoses, & provides treatment plan & documents accordingly

Superbill completed to include diagnosis & level of service provided

Patient Visit Completion Process:
Treatment plan reviewed & scheduling performed;
Financial responsibility addressed & managed;
Is a referral needed for additional treatments?
When discharging a patient, it is important to address question or concerns at that time; don't let your patient leave confused.
Remember it is your reputation. I have made customer service my practice platform.

SUPER BILL EXAMPLE

PATIENT NAME			DOB	AGE		COPAY	PREV. PERS. BALANCE		
PROVIDER			LOCATION	APPT TYPE		APPT DATE	APPT TIME		

	NEW PATIENT VISITS			ESTABLISHED VISITS		APPOINTMENT NEEDS			
99201	PROBLEM FOCUSED		99211	MINIMUM		FOLLOW UP			
99202	EXP/PROB FOCUSED		99212	PROBLEM FOCUSED					
99203	DETAILED		99213	EXP/PROB FOCUSED		DAILY	1 X 4	1 X 12	
99204	COMPREHENSIVE		99214	DETAILED		PT+ MANIP	PT ONLY	VAX-D	
CPT	Chiropractic Treatment	UNITS	CPT	DOCTOR MANUALS		REFER TO			
98940	1 TO 2 REGIONS		97140	GRASTON					
98941	3 TO 4 REGIONS		97110	ART		INJECTION	MEDS	CONSULTATION	
98942	EXTREMITY ADJUSTMENT		97139	TAPING		DIAGNOSTICS			
CPT	MODALITIES	UNITS	CPT	THERAPEUTIC	UNITS				
97010	HOT PACK		97140	MANUAL THERAPY		LABWORK	MRI	CT	EMG
97010	COLD PACK		97150	GROUP THERAPEUTIC ACT		CPT	RADIOLOGY		UNITS
97035	ULTRASOUND		97110	THERAPEUTIC PROCEDURE		72040	AP/LAT CERVICAL		
97012	TRACTION		97112	NEUROMUSCULAR RE-ED		72050	CERVICAL (4)		
G0283(WC)	E- STIMULATION		97116	GAIT TRAINING		72052	CERVICAL (7V)		
97139	SPRAY & STRETCH		97113	AQUATIC THERAPY		72100	AP/LAT LUMBAR		
CPT	WORK HARD & PREP	FEE	97535	ACTIVITIES DAILY LIVING		72110	LUMBAR OBLIQUE (2V)		
97545	WC (INITIAL 2 HRS)		97530	THERAPEUTIC ACTIVITIES		72070	AP/LAT THORACIC		
97546	WC (ADDL 2 HRS)		97113	AQUATIC THERAPY		73560	KNEE (2V)		
CPT	MISC SUPPLIES / CHARGES		CPT	MISC SUPPLIES/ CHARGES	FEE	73100	WRIST (2V)		
E0730	TENS UNIT PURCHASE	$50.00	A4556	ELECTRODES		73070	ELBOW (2V)		
64550	TENS UNIT APPLICATION		E1399	THERABAND		73030	SHOULDER (2V)		
L0140	CERVICAL COLLAR	$15.00		MIRACLE RUB/ BIOFREEZE	$10.00	73510	HIP (2V)		
L0500	LUMBAR CORSET	$35.00				73630	FOOT & ANKLE (2V)		

MUSCLES									
IT BAND	ERECTOR SPINAE	GLUTEUS	HAMSRINGS	HIP FLEXOR	ILIOCOSTALIS	LEVATOR	PARASPINAL	PIRIFORMIS	
PSOAS	RHOMBOID	SCALENES	SCM	SERRATUS	SPINALIS	SUBOCCIPITAL	TRAPEZIUS		

HX:

MODALITIES & REGION	STRETCHNG / ART / GRASTON	CHANGES
E/STIM ULTRASOUND MASSAGE (REG / ICE) TP RELEASE		IMPROVED : ROM FLEXIBILITY GAIT POSTURE
HEAT ICE CRYO-CRCULATOR		DECREASED: ROM FLEXIBILITY
OTHER:		OTHER:

THERAPY NOTES:

NOTES:

_____   _____
Doctor Signature   Therapist

BILLING & COLLECTIONS PROCESS TO ASSURE FINANCIAL SUCCESS

This area can be a little frustrating and hard to manage. Understand the billing and collection process to assure you are actually collecting every penny humanly possible. The billing/collections department of the practice is usually blamed for how the practice is doing; yet the truth is the financial billing department is the clean-up crew. Yes they collect – however, they collect what is given to them. What does this mean? It has to be right from the start; otherwise your team is chasing their tail trying to collect the money the practice deserves. This is the 3rd and 4th procedure required for financial success. Understanding all of the processes and owning responsibility in managing them will assure financial success.

BILLING OF SERVICES

FRONT OFFICE END OF DAY PROCESS

- Service is performed and Superbill/ Fee Slip is completed.
- Completed Fee Slip is turned into billing.
- Fee Slips reviewed for diagnosis and procedure codes.
- Fee Slips are verified against sign-in sheet to assure capture of all patient visits and services rendered.
- Once all Fee Slips are accounted for, they are submitted to Billing for processing.

BILLING DEPARTMENT PROCESS

- Fee Slips are entered into Practice Management Software, or reviewed if entered into EMR for accuracy. Corrections are made according to documentation or plan limits.

- Billing Report should then be run to verify billing.
    - Verify Diagnosis
    - Verify Procedure Codes and Modifiers
    - Verify the number of services billed against plan limits

- Once the Billing Report is verified, it may be sent through a Claim Scrubber and corrected accordingly.
    - A claims scrubber verifies demographic issues, coding issues, and diagnosis.

- Once Claims are clear through the Claim Scrubber, both electronic and paper claims are processed.

- The NEXT business day the submission report is worked.
    - Rejections or Claim Failures are corrected and resubmitted accordingly.

COLLECTIONS DEPARTMENT PROCESS

- Accounts Receivable Management Should Begin at Day 30 for Most Insurance Payers.

- W/C Claims are followed at Day 45 because Workers Compensation Carriers are allotted 45 days before status information is available.

- Carrier is called to verify Claim Status.
    - In processing - Follow up 10 days later.
    - Paid - Indicate paid date and follow-up in 10 days to assure payment is received.
    - Claim Not on File - Fax claim for processing - Follow up in 10 days.
    - Denied - Review the reason and appeal if necessary.

- Payments are Posted Daily for Accurate Accounts Receivable Management.

- Once Payment is Posted, Patient Collection begins.
    - Statement is sent weekly.
    - Outstanding patient portion is collected at the front desk.
    - Collections calls begin within 2 weeks if NO payment is received.
    - Manage the patient portion by offering payment plans, if necessary.
    - If a Patient Account reaches 120 days and no payment is received, the account is referred to a collection agency. We prefer soft collections (not placed on credit), but you will be surprised how many patients call to pay on their accounts when they get a collection letter from an agency.

Patient finances are a touchy subject in any practice. We have made it a policy to prohibit our providers from becoming involved in patient finances. Patient concerns are immediately referred to the Office Manger for resolution. Advise the patient that the doctor has made it a policy to be focused on patient care not their finances. This absolves the doctor from addressing the billing issue or becoming involved in something that can hurt your provider-patient relationship.

BILLING OF SERVICES CHART

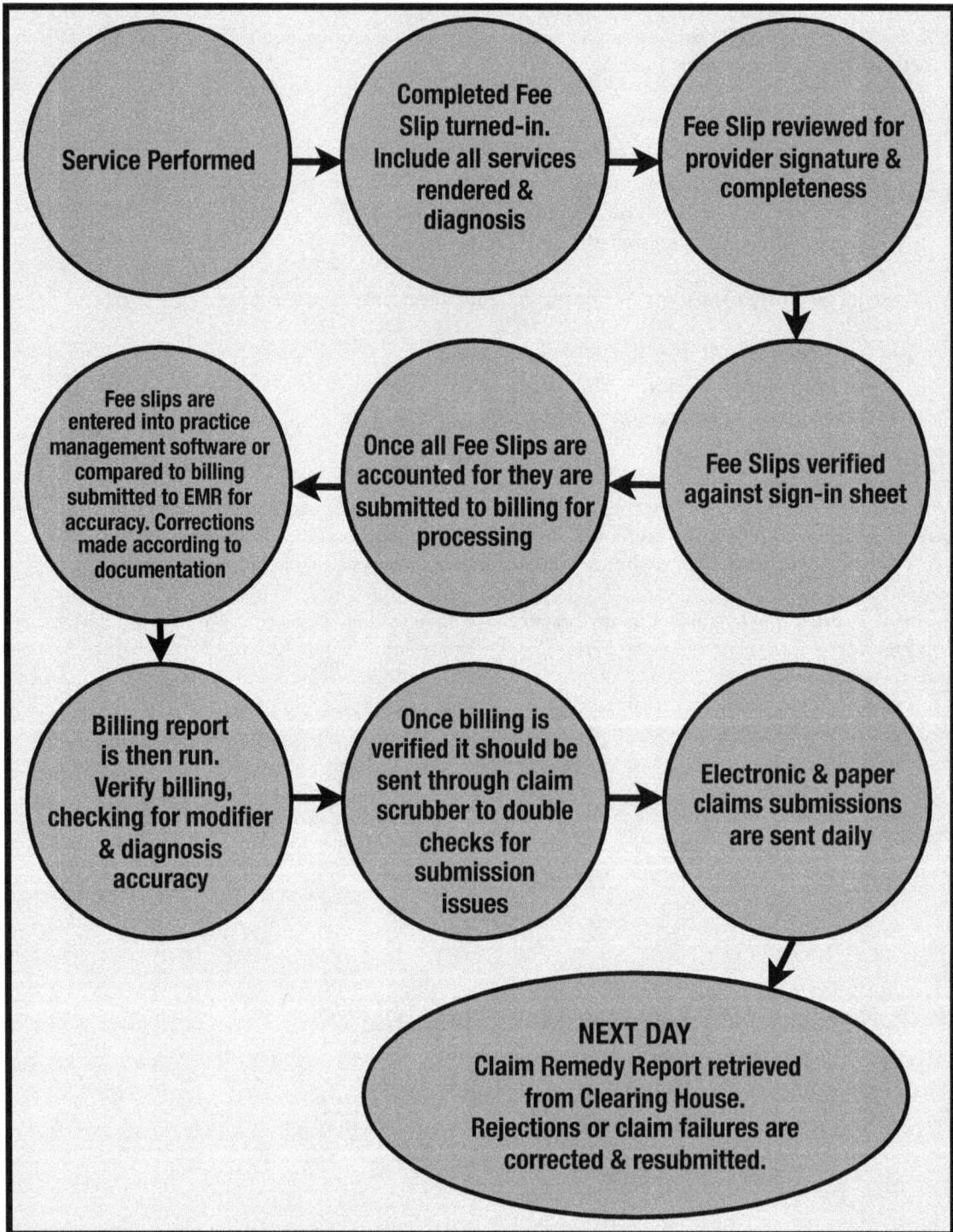

Service Performed

→

Completed Fee Slip turned-in. Include all services rendered & diagnosis

→

Fee Slip reviewed for provider signature & completeness

↓

Fee slips are entered into practice management software or compared to billing submitted to EMR for accuracy. Corrections made according to documentation

←

Once all Fee Slips are accounted for they are submitted to billing for processing

←

Fee Slips verified against sign-in sheet

↓

Billing report is then run. Verify billing, checking for modifier & diagnosis accuracy

→

Once billing is verified it should be sent through claim scrubber to double checks for submission issues

→

Electronic & paper claims submissions are sent daily

↓

NEXT DAY
Claim Remedy Report retrieved from Clearing House. Rejections or claim failures are corrected & resubmitted.

COLLECTION OF SERVICES RENDERED CHART

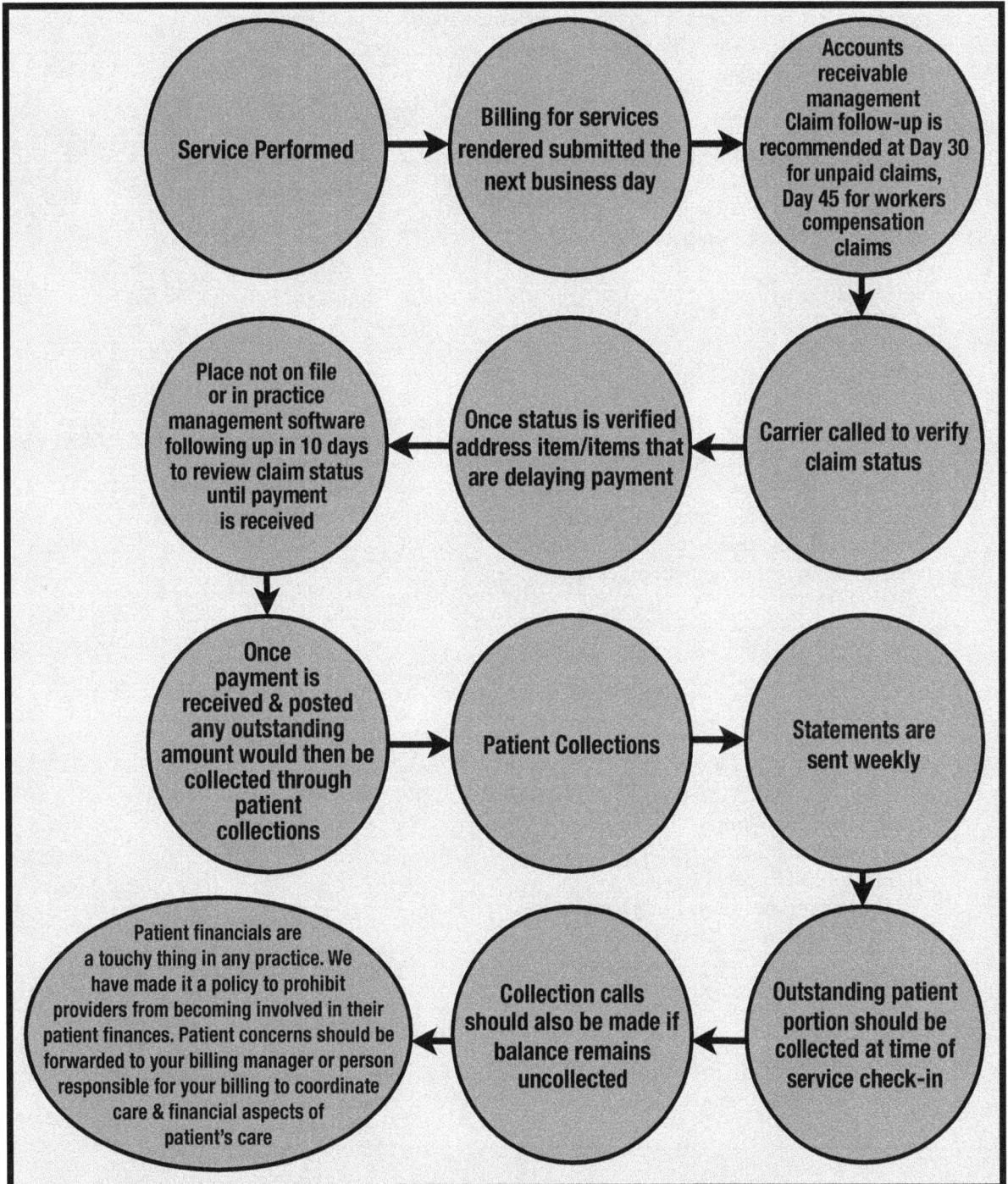

Service Performed → **Billing for services rendered submitted the next business day** → **Accounts receivable management Claim follow-up is recommended at Day 30 for unpaid claims, Day 45 for workers compensation claims**

Place not on file or in practice management software following up in 10 days to review claim status until payment is received ← **Once status is verified address item/items that are delaying payment** ← **Carrier called to verify claim status**

Once payment is received & posted any outstanding amount would then be collected through patient collections → **Patient Collections** → **Statements are sent weekly**

Patient financials are a touchy thing in any practice. We have made it a policy to prohibit providers from becoming involved in their patient finances. Patient concerns should be forwarded to your billing manager or person responsible for your billing to coordinate care & financial aspects of patient's care ← **Collection calls should also be made if balance remains uncollected** ← **Outstanding patient portion should be collected at time of service check-in**

E&M PATIENT CRITERIA

Coding for your services is critical in the fiscal stability of your practice. The outline below is a quick reference of the basic requirements to bill for the listed codes. The key to billing and being paid at the highest level is a complete understanding of the codes and the documentation requirement to support the billing for services rendered. Reimbursement is all about documentation, as insurance carriers request records and perform audits on a regular basis. This being said, knowledge is power.

Patient Type: New
- Description: New to group specialty within 3 years
  - No physician from same specialty in the same group
  - No professional services in the last 3 years
- Related E/M Codes for outpatient services
  - CPT 99201
  - CPT 99202
  - CPT 99203
  - CPT 99204
  - CPT 99205

Patient Type: Established
- Description: Care from group specialty within 3 years
  - Physician from same specialty in the same group
  - Professional services in the last 3 years
  - Includes call coverage
- Related E/M Codes for outpatient services
  - CPT 99211
  - CPT 99212
  - CPT 99213
  - CPT 99214
  - CPT 99215

New Outpatient: CPT Code 99201
- Key Components (All 3 meet or exceed requirements)
  Physician Time: 10 minutes
  - E/M Problem Focused History
  - E/M Problem Focused Exam
  - E/M Straightforward Medical Decision
  - E/M Self Limited or Minor Problem

Established Outpatient: CPT Code 99211
- Key components not required
  Staff Time: 5 minutes (Physician need not be present only supervising)
    - E/M Minimal Problem

New Outpatient: CPT Code 99202
- Key Components (All 3 meet or exceed requirements)
  Physician Time: 20 minutes
    - E/M Expanded Problem Focused History
    - E/M Expanded Problem Focused Exam
    - E/M Straightforward Medical Decision - Problem severity
    - E/M Low Severity Problem
    - E/M Moderate Severity Problem

Established Outpatient: CPT Code 99212
- Key Components (2 of 3 meet or exceed requirements)
  Physician Time: 10 minutes
    - E/M Problem Focused History
    - E/M Problem Focused Exam
    - E/M Straightforward Medical Decision
    - E/M Self Limited or Minor Problem

New Outpatient: CPT Code 99203
- Key Components (All 3 meet or exceed requirements)
  Physician Time: 30 minutes
    - E/M Detailed History
    - E/M Detailed Exam
    - E/M Low Complexity Medical Decision
    - E/M Moderate Severity Problem

Established Outpatient: CPT Code 99213
- Key Components (2 of 3 meet or exceed requirements)
  Physician Time: 15 minutes
    - E/M Expanded Problem Focused History
    - E/M Expanded Problem Focused Exam
    - E/M Low Complexity Medical Decision -Problem severity
    - E/M Low Severity Problem
    - E/M Moderate Severity Problem

New Outpatient: CPT Code 99204
- Key Components (All 3 meet or exceed requirements)
  Physician Time: 45 minutes
  - o E/M Comprehensive History
  - o E/M Comprehensive Exam
  - o E/M Moderate Complexity Medical Decision -Problem Severity
  - o E/M Moderate Severity Problem
  - o E/M High Severity Problem

Established Outpatient: CPT Code 99214
- Key Components (All 3 meet or exceed requirements)
  Physician Time: 30 minutes
  - o E/M Comprehensive History
  - o E/M Comprehensive Exam
  - o E/M Moderate Complexity Medical Decision -Problem Severity
  - o E/M Moderate Severity Problem
  - o E/M High Severity Problem

99212 VS. 99213

To begin, it is important to realize that you do not need to be presented with a complex or detailed problem in order to bill at the 99213. If a normally healthy patient sees you for a paper cut, it may be suitable to bill at the lower level. On the other hand, if the patient has some type of immune disorder, the cut is infected, or located near a finger joint, it would be better to bill at the higher code. In a similar way, visits for patients with stable, but chronic diabetes, hypertension, or obesity can usually be coded as 99213.

- When choosing between codes 99212 and 99213, be mindful of the amount of time spent with the patient, as well as any discussions about medical history. Anything that removes focus from the initial complaint can help with billing at the higher code. Among other things, if the patient starts talking about sinus problems, or family illness, document those facts in the chart. The additional diagnosis codes, plus medical history review will ensure that the criteria for billing at the higher level are met. Depending on the number of conditions discussed, the visit may actually qualify to be billed as a 99214.

- Article Source: http://EzineArticles.com/3640257

E/M CODE COMPARISON
ESTABLISHED PATIENT

ESTABLISHED PATIENT VISITS: CPT codes & documentation requirements	E/M CODE				
	99211	99212	99213	99214	99215
HISTORY					
Chief Complaint	Required	Required	Required	Required	Required
History of present illness	NR	1-3 elements	1-3 elements	≥4 elements or ≥3 chronic diseases	≥4 elements or ≥3 chronic diseases
Review of systems	NR	NR	1 system	2-9 systems	≥10 systems
Past history/family history & social history	NR	NR	NR	1 element	≥2 elements
EXAMINATION	NR	1 brief system (1-5 elements)	2 brief systems (6-11 elements)	1 detailed system + 1 brief system (≥2 elements)	8 systems or 1 complete single system (comprehensive)
MEDICAL DECISION MAKING					
Risk	NR	Minimal	Low	Moderate	High
Diagnosis or treatment options	Minimal	Minimal	Low	Moderate	High
Data	NR	Minimal	Low/Moderate	Moderate	High
Time*	5 minutes	10 minutes	15 minutes	25 minutes	40 minutes

CPT, current procedural terminology, E/M, evaluation & management, HPI, history of presenting illness, NR, not required
*At least one half of total face-to-face time must involve counseling or coordination of care.
Adapted from: American Medical Association

E/M CODE COMPARISON

NEW PATIENT

NEW PATIENT VISIT: CPT codes & documentation requirements	E/M CODE				
	99201	**99202**	**99203**	**99204**	**99205**
HISTORY					
Chief Complaint	Required	Required	Required	Required	Required
History of present illness	1-3 elements	1-3 elements	≥4 elements or ≥3 chronic diseases	≥4 elements or ≥3 chronic diseases	≥4 elements or ≥3 chronic diseases
Review of systems	NR	1 system	2 systems	≥10 systems	≥10 systems
Past history/family history & social history	NR	NR	1 element	≥3 elements	≥3 elements
EXAMINATION	1 system (1-5 elements)	2 brief systems (6-11 elements)	1 detailed system + 1 brief system (≥12 elements)	8 systems or 1 complete single system (comprehensive)	8 systems or 1 complete single system (comprehensive)
MEDICAL DECISION MAKING					
Risk	NR	Minimal	Low	Moderate	High
Diagnosis or treatment options	Minimal	Minimal	Low	Moderate	High
Data	Minimal	Minimal	Low	Moderate	High
Time*	10 minutes	20 minutes	30 minutes	45 minutes	60 minutes

CPT, current procedural terminology, E/M, evaluation & management, HPI, history of presenting illness, NR, not required
At least one half of total face-to-face time must involve counseling or coordination of care.
Adapted from: American Medical Association

DOCUMENT AND BILL MORE 99214s

Centers for Medicare & Medicaid Services (CMS) data show that in 2006, family physicians billed 55.2% of their established outpatient visits as level 3s (99213) and 31.6% as level 4s (99214).2 Evidence suggests that the percentage of 99214s could legitimately be higher. A study comparing family physicians' choice of codes with those selected by expert coders revealed that the physicians under-coded one third (1/3) of their established patient visits. In most cases, visits that warranted 99214 codes were instead coded as 99213s.

To bill for a level 4 established patient visit, CPT (Current Procedural Terminology) guidelines require the fulfillment of 2 out of 3 of the following components:

- A Detailed History
- A Detailed Physical Examination
- Medical Decision Making Of Moderate Complexity

FAST TRACK

Be aware of the tendency to code according to the complexity of the diagnosis, rather than the extent of decision making involved.

When the history and medical decision making indicate a higher level of complexity, you can bill for a 99214 visit without having to count or document individual body systems or detailed exam elements. A new diagnosis with a prescription, an order for laboratory tests or X-rays, or requests for a specialty consult are all examples of moderately complex decision making. When it is necessary to show that you performed a comprehensive system review to justify a 99214 claim, history forms, filled out in the waiting room and subsequently reviewed.

THERAPY CODE TIME REQUIREMENTS

- **97010** Hot & Cold Packs - Application of a modality to one or more areas. No time requirement

- **S9090** Mechanical Traction - This code stands alone and can only be billed once daily

- **G0283/97014** Electrical Stimulation Unattended- The G0283 has primarily replaced code 97014 with most insurance carriers. This code is a timed code for each 15 minutes.

- **97035** Ultrasound - Application of a modality to one or more areas; each 15 minutes

- **97110** Therapeutic procedure, one or more areas, each 15 minutes; therapeutic exercises to develop strength and endurance, range of motion and flexibility

- **97112** Neuromuscular Re-education of movement, one or more areas, each 15 minutes; balance, coordination, kinesthetic sense, posture, and/or proprioception for sitting and/or standing activities

- **97116** Gait Training - one or more areas, each 15 minutes; (includes stair climbing)

- **97140** Manual therapy techniques (e.g., mobilization/ manipulation, manual lymphatic drainage, manual traction), one or more regions, each 15 minutes.
  - 97140 Manual therapy techniques consist of, but are not limited to, connective tissue massage, joint mobilization and manipulation, manual traction, passive range of motion, soft tissue mobilization and manipulation, and therapeutic massage including manual lymphatic drainage, one or more regions, each 15 minutes. Code 97140 is time-based - not diagnosis or region-based. The Physical Medicine section of Current Procedural Terminology (CPT) identifies 97140 as a constant attendance code, meaning that it requires direct one-to-one patient contact by the provider. Time-based means that the service is billable in 15-minute increments, called units. Timeframes include all the work for pre-service, intra-service, and post-service.

- **97530** Therapeutic Activities-Direct one to one patient contact by the provider (use of dynamic activities to improve functional performance) each 15 minutes.

- **97535** Activities Of Daily Living –self-care/home-management training (such as ADL and compensatory training, meal preparation, safety procedures, and instructions in the use of assistive technology devices/adaptive equipment) with direct, one-on-one contact by the provider, each 15 minutes.
  - This should be reported for the provider/therapist devoting a separate and distinct procedural service to the patient for the purpose of instructing the patient in managing an injury at home and preventing a secondary injury, and instructing the patient on how to prevent future exacerbations.

THERAPY TIME DELINEATION

Time intervals for one through four units are as follows:

- One unit: eight minutes through 22 minutes,
- Two units: 23 minutes through 37 minutes,
- Three units: 38 minutes through 52 minutes, and
- Four units: 53 minutes through 67 minutes.

* If a service represented by a 15-minute timed code is performed in a single day for at least 15 minutes, that service can be billed for at least one unit. If the service is performed for at least 30 minutes, that service can be billed for at least two units, etc.

CMT CODING LEVELS

CMT coding usually can not be combined with an E & M code.

There are exceptions to this rule as follows:

- Adjusting the Spinal Region and addressing another diagnosis outside the area of adjustment.
- An acute exacerbation with a change in treatment plan.
- Using an E&M code and a CMT code will almost always delay payment and require records.
  * Documentation is the key.

MANIPULATION

- 98940 – Chiropractic Manipulative Treatment - Spinal 1-2 regions
- 98941 – Chiropractic Manipulative Treatment - Spinal 3-4 regions
- 98942 – Chiropractic Manipulative Treatment - 5 Spinal regions
- 98943 – Chiropractic Manipulative Treatment – Extra-Spinal 1 or more Regions

SPINAL REGIONS OF MANIPULATION

- Cervical Region
- Lumbar Region
- Pelvic Region
- Sacral Region
- Thoracic Region

EXTRASPINAL REGIONS OF MANIPULATION

- Abdomen
- Head, including temporomandibular joint, excluding atlanto-occipital region
- Lower Extremities
- Rib Cage, not including costotransverse/costovertebral joints
- Upper Extremities
  o 98942- Extremity Adjustment Code

PATIENT EDUCATION

PATIENT EDUCATION

- Patient education begins the initial day the patient arrives. During the evaluation, explain to the patient the treating order of "the boxes" and the need to treat accordingly.

- Provide educational sheets along with Home Exercise Plans if applicable.

- Explain importance of using injections to decrease inflammation quickly and progress rehabilitation and promote healing.

- Educate regarding the benefits of monthly adjustments. Once a Patient is at a manageable level, they transition to monthly visits.

PATIENT WARNING SIGNS

1. Weakness of Face, Arm, or Leg
   - Especially on One Side of The Body

2. Sudden Confusion

3. Trouble Speaking or Understanding

4. Trouble Seeing in One or Both Eyes

5. Trouble Walking

6. Dizziness, Loss of Balance or Coordination

7. Sudden or Severe Headache

8. Chest Pains

9. Severe, Uncontrolled Pain

10. Fainting

11. Convulsions

International Health Publishing

Inspiring readers of the world to experience the light.

International Health Publishing books express truth and wisdom, encourage spiritual enlightenment, facilitate growth and healing – while also providing a phenomenal reading experience.

International Health Publishing's vision is to increase the number and quality of books and resources available to the public, students and Doctors of Chiropractic – allowing for greater understanding, increased education, as well as more visibility and accessibility of the Chiropractic profession as a means of preventative and continued health care.

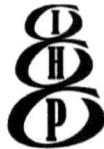

International Health Publishing

Adjusting and Growing

International Headquarters • Carrollton, Texas

www.InternationalHealthPublishing.com

www.ingramcontent.com/pod-product-compliance
Lightning Source LLC
Chambersburg PA
CBHW080244270326
41926CB00020B/4372

* 9 7 8 0 9 8 5 7 9 5 6 8 9 *